The
Appetite
Solution

The Appetite Solution

Lose Weight Effortlessly
and Never Be Hungry Again

613.25

Joe Colella, M.D.

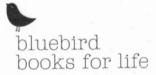

bluebird
books for life

First published 2015 by HarperOne, an imprint of HarperCollins Publishers

First published in the UK 2015 by Bluebird
an imprint of Pan Macmillan, a division of Macmillan Publishers Limited
Pan Macmillan, 20 New Wharf Road, London N1 9RR
Basingstoke and Oxford
Associated companies throughout the world
www.panmacmillan.com

ISBN 978-1-5098-0234-0

This book is intended as a reference volume only, not as a medical manual. The information
given here is designed to help you make informed decisions about your health. It is not
intended as a substitute for any treatment that you may have been prescribed by your doctor.
If you suspect you have a medical problem, we urge you to seek competent medical help.

Mention of specific companies, organizations or authorities in this book does not imply
endorsement of the publisher, nor does mention of specific companies, organizations
or authorities in the book imply that they endorse the book. Addresses, websites and
telephone numbers given in this book were correct at the time of going to press.

Macmillan does not have any control over, or any responsibility for,
any author or third party websites referred to in or on this book.

9 8 7 6 5 4 3 2 1

A CIP catalogue record for this book is available from the British Library.

Designed by Ruth Lee-Mui
Printed and bound by CPI Group (UK) Ltd, Croydon, CR0 4YY

Visit **www.panmacmillan.com** to read more about all our books and to buy them.
You will also find features, author interviews and news of any author events, and you
can sign up for e-newsletters so that you're always first to hear about our new releases.

To my glorious sons Joey and Luke. No father could be more blessed.

Contents

I'm Always Hungry, and I Can't Lose Weight

It's January 2 and Naomi is ready to start keeping her most important New Year's resolution: *Go on a diet and lose weight!* She'd like fast results to keep her motivated, so she picks a low-carbohydrate diet that a friend has recommended, one that has her cutting her food intake to 1,000 calories a day. Just as her friend has told her, Naomi loses ten pounds (4.5 kilos) in two weeks, and she is ecstatic.

Of course, she's hungry all the time—but she knows the weight loss will be worth it, and with an iron will, she sticks to every detail of the diet. When the two weeks are over, the diet plan becomes less restrictive, and Naomi breathes a sigh of relief. But she's still always hungry; and then, suddenly, she stops losing weight.

Frustrated and disappointed, Naomi toughs it out on this new diet for another few weeks but then finally gives up in despair. She goes back to eating the way she did before, continues to feel hungry—and by April 1, she is actually five pounds (2.25 kilos) heavier than she was on January 1.

Shana also has a New Year's resolution to keep—in fact, it's almost the same as Naomi's: *Start a diet and fitness plan and lose weight!* Shana normally consumes about 2,000 calories a day, so she goes on a low-fat diet that is somewhat less restrictive than Naomi's—down to 1,500 calories. At the same time, she joins a gym, signs up with a personal trainer, and begins a vigorous fitness program.

Shana notices that she, too, is hungry all the time, but during her first week on the diet, she loses five pounds (2.25 kilos), which motivates her to keep going. A few days later, however, she hits a hard plateau and the weight loss grinds to a halt.

Frustrated and hungry, Shana cuts her calories back to 1,300 per day and steps up the exercise. She manages to lose another two pounds (barely a kilo)—and then, again, a plateau. Her fitness instructor encourages her to tough it out, but the following week, Shana has actually started to gain back some of the weight she's lost. By April 1, she is just about three pounds (1.4 kilos) less than the weight at which she started her diet and exercise plan, and she's more frustrated and hungrier than ever.

Greg would also like to lose weight, so on January 2, he works with a nutritionist to follow a super-healthy diet with lots of fresh fruits and vegetables, no grains, and no starches—about 2,000 calories a day. He hasn't been able to make time for exercise, but his nutritionist assures him that this diet will work if Greg sticks to it faithfully.

For breakfast, Greg enjoys a protein shake with fresh blueberries buzzed in, or perhaps a hard-boiled egg and a glass of freshly squeezed orange juice. For lunch, he eats a salad with salmon or turkey and low-fat dressing. For his afternoon snack, he has a fat-free vanilla yogurt and a skimmed decaf latte. For dinner, he grills some chicken with barbecue sauce or simmers it in some of his mum's homemade tomato sauce and steams up a big bowl of broccoli. All day long he drinks water flavored with a couple of lemon wedges, or maybe has some decaf coffee with fat-free coffee creamer.

Greg began this diet on January 2, and he sticks it to faithfully every day, never exceeding his allotted 2,000 calories. By April 1, he's lost just over three pounds (1.4 kilos), most of which he dropped during the first month. To make matters worse, he feels hungry all the time. What's going wrong?

Do any of these scenarios sound familiar to you? Have you been starving yourself on a diet, running yourself ragged at the gym, or eating an apparently healthy diet, yet you either can't lose weight or can't keep the weight off—plus you're hungry all the time? Have you been blaming the problem on your lack of willpower? Your "fat genes"? Your "big bones"?

Your lifelong lousy metabolism? Does it sometimes feel like you're the victim of a conspiracy to keep you overweight and hungry?—that everywhere you look you see desirable food you're not supposed to eat, and yet even when you resist it, your weight stays on?

Believe me, I understand. I've helped thousands of people who feel exactly the same way dealing every day with hunger and frustration. I know I can help you, too. I'm going to show you how to beat each of these scenarios—how to lose your excess weight and keep it off, *without being hungry.*

Does that sound too good to be true? I promise you, it *is* true. The Appetite Solution can be *your* solution: steady, significant weight loss without feeling hungry, until you ultimately achieve the metabolism of a teenager. You can keep eating many of your favorite foods, you'll never feel like you're starving, and when you do achieve a teenager's high-powered metabolism, you can even indulge periodically in some missed treats.

If that sounds good to you, stick with me. Let's start by taking a closer look at why so many diets fail.

A Dieter's Three Pitfalls

Three major pitfalls prevail with dieters, and most people fall into one, two, or all three:

- ☐ They begin a diet by cutting calories, and by default, their protein intake.
- ☐ They start a diet and a fitness program at the same time.
- ☐ They don't know how to recognize *simple sugars*, especially the hidden ones, versus *complex sugars*, which occur naturally in fruits, vegetables, and grains.

Naomi, Shana, and Greg each fell into a different pitfall, but they all had one thing in common: *Each of their diets left them feeling hungry.*

In the world of dieting, that should be your first clue:

> Any diet that leaves you feeling constantly hungry is almost certainly doomed to fail.

Why do I say this? Well, first, of course, the hunger often means that you simply can't stay on the diet. It's very difficult to keep denying yourself the foods you enjoy in the face of a punishing hunger—especially if you're not losing weight.

But even if you do stick to your plan, a diet that leaves you hungry is messing with your metabolism. Anything more than a mild hunger after the first two or three days of a diet is a sign that a process known as *adaptive thermogenesis* has kicked in. *And adaptive thermogenesis is going to make it virtually impossible for you to lose weight.* It always wins.

The Perils of Adaptive Thermogenesis

Adaptive thermogenesis is the mechanism that your body has evolved to keep from starving to death or wasting away when you can't get enough to eat or have to exert yourself more than usual. *Adaptive* refers to something that has adapted in response to circumstances. *Thermo* means "heat," that is, energy, or calories. *Genesis* comes from the Latin for "generation"; so thermogenesis is the generation, or production, of heat in the body.

Put that all together, and adaptive thermogenesis means that when your body perceives that you aren't getting your usual amount of food, for example, on your brand-new diet, it will do everything in its power to adapt by conserving energy—to *stop* burning calories and to force you to seek out more calories. Likewise, when your body perceives that you are exerting yourself more than usual, for example, with your brand-new fitness program, it will again adapt to conserve energy, ensuring that your new vigorous activity burns as few calories as possible.

Note that adaptive thermogenesis kicks in when you aren't getting your *usual* amount of food and when you are exercising more than *usual.* That's what makes it adaptive. Even if you are switching from an unhealthy level of calorie intake to a healthier one, even if you are finally getting some much-needed healthy exercise, your body still responds ("adapts") to the *change,* not to the absolute level of your diet or activity.

As a result, any decline in calories and any increase in exercise sends your body straight into panic mode, terrified of starvation or exhaustion.

Adaptive thermogenesis always does its darnedest to hold on to every last bit of weight.

Now at this point you might be wondering: "Then why does my diet seem to work at the beginning? How did I lose those first few pounds or kilos?"

Great questions. Although some diets, like Greg's, never do get going (and in a minute I'll tell you why), Naomi and Shana *did* lose weight initially, even though they gained some of it back or hit a plateau fairly early, after only a small loss. Why?

Well, here's the dirty little secret that most diet books won't tell you. That initial lost weight is almost always *muscle mass* and the water that goes with it. Cutting calories and starting a diet-plus-fitness plan at the same time does not induce your body to get rid of fat—instead, it causes you to lose muscle.

Don't Let Your Body Eat Itself for Breakfast!

Most of us think of "losing weight" as "losing fat"—but that's not what happens when you are hungry. Eating a low-calorie diet might help you shed a little weight initially, but when your body thinks it's starving, fat is the last thing to go.

Maybe you, in your twenty-first-century culture of plenty, would like to lose those extra fatty layers, but your ancestors, back in the hard times, clung to that fat for dear life—literally. Body fat kept those ancestors warm. Body fat was a source of stored energy. Body fat was what a woman needed in order to menstruate and to get pregnant and to carry a child. Body fat was what people lived on all winter long.

Muscle, by contrast, is a luxury. Yeah, muscles are nice for pushing boulders and chopping trees and other types of vigorous activity. But if food is scarce, you don't want to be burning up calories running around exerting yourself. You want to *conserve* energy, not expend it. If your body believes that it isn't getting enough food, it would much rather eat up its muscle than burn off its fat. So when you start most diets, that's exactly what it does, devouring muscle to make up the difference between the amount of calories you *usually* eat and the amount you just started eating.

So after your first week on a reduced-calorie diet, you look at the scale and think, "Great! I lost five pounds (2.25 kilos)!" You don't realize that that was the five pounds (2.25 kilos) of muscle which your *body* ate to compensate for the food that *you* didn't eat, plus the water that your muscle contained.

Then, within ten to fourteen days, adaptive thermogenesis helps your body reset. It jiggers your metabolism to burn fewer calories with the same amount of exercise and to hold on to more calories with the same amount of food. At this point, you're still eating up your own muscles even though you're not losing weight. Your body is keeping things as much the same as possible, using your muscles to make up for any reduction in calories. It's an ingenious system, and it might have saved your life back in the Stone Age, but it can sure drive you crazy now.

This is why I say that hunger should be your first clue that a diet isn't working. Hunger is a sign that adaptive thermogenesis is at work, ensuring the following outcomes:

☐ You will initially lose some weight as your body consumes some of its own muscle and the water it contains.

☐ You will eventually remain at a steady weight, *no matter how little you eat or how much you exercise,* as your body figures out new ways to conserve energy. In fact, if you restrict your calories *more* and ramp up the exercise *further,* you might make it even *harder* to lose weight because your body will be even more alarmed and will work even harder to prevent that. Your hunger will increase—but your fat will not disappear (though some more muscle might).

Eventually, as Naomi found, you might experience a third outcome that is even less desirable than the other two:

☐ You will *gain* weight because you have started to eat a bit more than you did on your restrictive diet—but now your metabolism has been reset down to "low intake," so it uses those extra calories to store some extra fat.

We'll learn more about adaptive thermogenesis in chapter 1, along with another fat-storing trigger—stress. Any time your body is stressed, it thinks,

"Starvation!" and a whole cascade of stress hormones join forces to incite fat storage. And guess what? Cutting calories is a stressor, and so is a new fitness program, and so is unquenchable hunger itself. Once again, persistent hunger is your danger signal, letting you know that your current approach to diet is *not working*.

That's not a danger signal you will get while following the Appetite Solution. Because I've been working nonstop with overweight and obese people for the past two decades, I know exactly what prevents weight loss—and what enables it. I have figured out how to foil adaptive thermogenesis, with an approach that no other published weight-loss program has yet tried, but which I have used successfully with countless patients. And I have made sure that from the morning of Day 4—and for many of you, even earlier—you will never feel more than a mild, pleasant hunger every four to five hours—exactly when it's time for your next meal.

> After the first two or three days, hunger is a danger signal. Any diet that causes you to be more than mildly hungry beyond that point is inciting adaptive thermogenesis and stress—both of which cue your body to hold on to fat.

The Sugar Saboteurs

I'm going to share my secret weapon with you in just a minute—the nutritional strategy I have developed to foil adaptive thermogenesis. But first, I want to point out that there is another reason you might be excessively hungry—long before the next meal, too soon after the last meal, or maybe even all day long. Greg ran into this pitfall on his supposedly healthy diet, for a very common reason: his diet contained far too many simple sugars.

When I explain this to people who are living on salad greens and salmon, they look at me in bewilderment, unsure whether I'm teasing them, have misunderstood, or maybe have just gone off the deep end.

But I'm dead serious: Greg's apparently healthy diet was full of simple sugars. Here are just some of the places that Greg was running into trouble:

- ☐ 1 cup (125 grams) blueberries blended into a shake: only 83 calories . . . but 15 grams of simple sugar.
- ☐ 8 ounces (230 grams) freshly squeezed orange juice: only 112 calories . . . but 21 grams of simple sugar.
- ☐ 1 tablespoon fat-free coffee creamer: only 35 calories . . . but 5 grams of simple sugar. (And *nobody* sticks to just 1 tablespoon.)
- ☐ 2 tablespoons fat-free French dressing: only 45 calories . . . but 5 grams of simple sugar. (And again, *nobody* sticks to just 2 tablespoons.)
- ☐ 1 cup (240 millilitres) tomato sauce: only 90 calories . . . but 10 grams of simple sugar.
- ☐ 1 tablespoon barbecue sauce: only 29 calories . . . but 5 grams of simple sugar. (And again: One tablespoon? Come on! Have you *seen* 1 tablespoon? If you're spreading that sauce over a whole breast of chicken, you've got to be using at least 4 tablespoons, which contain 20 grams of simple sugars.)

Now, guess how many grams of simple sugar are in a Cadbury's Mini Roll? Only 14. Even before he went on his healthy diet, Greg would never have dreamed of eating a mini roll. Yet every night that he slathered barbecue sauce on his skinless breast of chicken, he might as well have been doing just that.

If Greg had eaten his blueberries and his orange whole, by the way, and if he had grilled some fresh tomatoes or maybe sautéed them lightly, he would have been fine, for reasons that I'll explain in chapter 2. But Greg, like most dieters, had no idea that simple sugars lurk in so many seemingly healthy foods, nor that food preparation can make such a difference in how many grams of sugar are released and therefore easily available to be digested, absorbed, and released into your bloodstream. In chapter 2, I'll show you why the simple sugars in Greg's diet kept him perpetually hungry—and why they kept him perpetually overweight. Then, in chapter 3, I'll help you become a sugar detective so that you can locate all the different places simple sugars might be hiding, and I'll offer you some easy substitutions so that you can limit those simple sugars and rely more on complex sugars.

Okay, so cutting calories, starting a diet and fitness program at the same time, and failing to recognize simple sugars: those are the factors that invoke adaptive thermogenesis, inflate your appetite, threaten your muscle, and keep you from losing fat. But if they are the problems, what is the solution?

Announcing the Appetite Solution

My secret weapon is the Appetite Solution, a nutritional strategy guaranteed to make this eating plan work for you. Here is the element that will help you build lean muscle, let go of excess fat, transform your appetite, and, ultimately, help you achieve the metabolism of a teenager:

> → Ramp up the protein.

Protein, as you'll learn in chapter 1, has the extraordinary ability to jam the hunger signals that come at you from a dozen different places: not just the way simple sugars mess with your metabolism and your blood sugar levels, but also the effects of stress, lack of sleep, many medications, heartburn, anxiety, and depression. All of these factors inflate your appetite. Increasing the amount of protein you eat every day jams those signals at your brain.

To make matters worse, these signals don't just make you hungry—they make you ravenous for simple sugars. And simple sugars, as you'll learn in chapter 2, generate an insulin response that perpetually guarantees fat storage, weight gain, and a host of other problems.

So how do we keep you from craving simple sugars? By loading you up with protein.

Increasing your protein intake is going to make an enormous difference in transforming your appetite. It's also going to help you build lean muscle mass, which, as you'll see in chapter 1, has a powerful metabolic effect of its own, helping you to burn calories as soon as you consume them. My strategic use of protein is a big part of what will eventually enable you to achieve the metabolism of a teenager so that you have the license to indulge in a few treats.

Protein will help you circumvent the powerful effects of adaptive thermogenesis, but I want to go even further to persuade your body that it has nothing to fear. "Don't worry," I want to say to your metabolism. "We're not cutting calories. We're not increasing exertion. We're not doing anything that should provoke you to reset and hold on to fat." So here is the second principle of the Appetite Solution:

> → Cut simple sugars *without* immediately cutting calories.

Yes, you will eventually end up cutting calories. Actually, you will let go of them on your own, painlessly and of your own free will. But the initial focus won't be on calories at all. That's because all calories are not created equal. As you'll see in chapter 2, if you're on a diet that has you eating a 216-calorie cup (200 grams) of cooked brown rice, and you decide to skip the brown rice and eat a 113-calorie biscuit, you would obviously be choosing to eat fewer calories. But the brown rice has only 0.7 grams of simple sugars, while the biscuit has 9 grams.

What this means is that even though the brown rice has almost twice as many calories than the biscuit, the biscuit has a disastrous effect on your metabolism, while the brown rice causes no problems at all.

Why? All those simple sugars in the biscuit incite your pancreas to release *insulin,* the hormone that your body uses to move sugar from your blood into your cells. The more sugars that hit your bloodstream at one time, the more insulin your pancreas releases. And guess what insulin does besides move blood sugar into cells? It cues your body to store fat. You'll learn more about this process in chapter 2, but here's a simple diagram to make it clear:

> Simple sugars → insulin → fat storage
> (and this effect lingers long after you eat).

Notice that the word "calories" doesn't appear anywhere in that diagram. That's why my first concern for the Appetite Solution is not calories—it's simple sugars, the ones that evoke the biggest insulin response.

Many types of calories—such as those found in protein, fats, and complex carbohydrates—don't have the same metabolic effect as simple sugars. Proteins and fats don't evoke much of an insulin response at all. Complex carbs do, but very slowly, mildly, and in a delayed fashion. Only *simple* sugars incite your pancreas to flood your body with insulin—the insulin that in turn instructs your body to store fat. So in chapter 2, I'll explain to you exactly what the difference is between complex carbs and simple sugars, and in chapter 3, I'll teach you how to find simple sugars in all their clever hiding places.

Meanwhile, here's your takeaway:

☐ Because it contains so many simple sugars, the biscuit will mess with your blood sugar, your insulin levels, and your metabolism, keeping you overweight and hungry.

☐ Because it contains so few simple sugars, the higher-calorie bowl of brown rice—even if you soaked it in 2 or 3 tablespoons of butter—will do significantly less damage to your weight and far more to stabilize your appetite.

This brings us to the next principle of the Appetite Solution:

> → *When your body is ready,* you will limit yourself to 5 grams of simple sugars per meal and a total of 20 grams of simple sugars per day.

If I had you doing this from Day 1, you'd be climbing the walls by Day 4. It's hard to immediately cut out simple sugars, and I don't want this eating plan to be hard for you, because hard diets just don't work. Not to mention that I've just been telling you that hunger, stress, and an extreme reaction to cutting something out of your diet are all antithetical to the kind of weight loss you want.

So I *won't* be cutting simple sugars drastically on Day 1. Instead, I'll be cutting them very slowly while I nourish you with protein. For the first two weeks, I'll have you *slowly* and *gradually* cut back on simple sugars. Then, in Week 3, you'll be ready to cut simple sugars more aggressively. And by Week 5, you'll be on a low-simple-sugar plan that will enable fast, hunger-free weight loss.

And now we're ready for the final principle of the Appetite Solution:

> → Add in some vigorous, muscle-building exercise—*after* you've had sufficient protein intake without calorie reduction.

By the time you start exercising—in Week 3—you'll have a lot of protein in your diet, which will help foil adaptive thermogenesis. That protein tells your body, "Don't worry, you're not starving—no need to start eating yourself for breakfast." Your body also uses that protein to protect and build muscle. Meanwhile, cutting back on sugar reduces the insulin in your system, so your body can begin to burn fat and stop storing it on your hips.

The Appetite Solution at a Glance

Phase 1: Push the Protein, Weeks 1 and 2
- ☐ Ramp up your intake of protein.
- ☐ Slowly, gradually, begin to cut back on simple sugars.

Phase 2: Shelve the Sugar, Weeks 3 and 4
- ☐ Continue to consume a high level of protein.
- ☐ More aggressively lower your simple sugars until you reach their healthiest level.
- ☐ Begin a moderate exercise program as described in chapter 7.

Phase 3: Shed the Fat, Weeks 5 and 6 . . . and until you've reached your target weight
- ☐ Continue to consume a high level of protein.
- ☐ Keep simple sugar consumption at its lowest, healthiest level.
- ☐ Continue a moderate exercise program.

You've seen what happens with diets during which you shed weight quickly—they're usually inducing you to lose muscle, not fat. I don't want that to happen to you when you are following the Appetite Solution, so I'm not trying to get you to shed much weight early in the process.

However, you will lose *some* weight over the first month, and weight loss will pick up quickly after that. During Phase 3, you will lose three to five pounds (about 1.5 to 2 kilos) each week. And by the end of the six weeks of the Appetite Solution, you are likely to have lost fifteen pounds (close to 7 kilos) or half your excess weight, whichever is smaller.

In other words, by the end of Phase 3, you have hit the weight-loss home run: You have foiled adaptive thermogenesis. You have successfully put yourself on a hunger-free, sustainable, healthy weight-loss path—building muscle, burning fat—and you are well on your way to achieving the metabolism of a teenager.

No Deprivation!

One of the great things about the Appetite Solution is that you never have to feel deprived. Cutting simple sugars doesn't mean you have to cut complex carbs, and so you will enjoy a lot of healthy choices: wholemeal bread, whole-wheat pasta, whole grains like brown rice and quinoa, and sweet potatoes. You can even have porridge, as long as you don't throw in the wrong "extras" (don't worry, I'll guide you through!). Over time, you might find yourself eating less of these complex carbs, but you'll do so gradually and naturally, without ever feeling hungry.

You will also enjoy a lot of delicious healthy fats: olive oil, avocado, nuts, unsweetened nut butters, even regular butter. These will help keep you feeling full and satisfied—and all that healthy fat is good for every single cell in your body, especially your brain cells. Eating in a way that is based on the Appetite Solution, you will feel sharper and more focused than you have in a while, as well as calmer, more energized, and more optimistic.

"This Won't Work Because . . ."

As you've been reading, has one or more of the following thoughts been running through your mind?

- ☐ "I have bad genes."
- ☐ "I have a sweet tooth."
- ☐ "I've always been like this."
- ☐ "I have no willpower."

- ☐ "I have no discipline."
- ☐ "I have big bones."
- ☐ "I'm fine most of the time, but then a crisis happens and I'm back to wolfing down pasta and desserts."
- ☐ "I've been on every diet on the planet and none of them has ever worked for me."

Believe me, I get it. If you're like most of my patients, you've been dieting most of your life and you're running out of faith that you can *ever* lose the weight you want to get rid of, let alone keep it off, or even be able to stop feeling hungry. Or perhaps you're shocked at the way your weight seems to have ballooned up out of nowhere, after years of being able to remain at your ideal weight or at an "acceptable" few pounds or kilos extra.

Maybe your weight gain erupted after a life crisis, such as losing a job, going through a bad breakup, or caring for a sick parent. If you're a woman, maybe you've had children and haven't been able to lose the weight you gained during pregnancy. Maybe you've always been able to indulge, gain weight, and then lose it again—and now, suddenly, you can't lose any more.

And so now, you might even be starting to hate your body for making you feel so hungry all the time. Maybe you blame yourself. Perhaps you've begun to wonder which unresolved issues are driving your "stress eating" or "emotional eating." Or maybe you're just sick and tired of always being hungry.

I know it's hard to have faith when so many diets have already disappointed you, and I know it's hard not to blame yourself. But I'm speaking to you as a physician with decades of dealing with weight problems, and I'm here to tell you: You *can* lose weight and transform your appetite. You just need to do it with an eating plan that doesn't leave you hungry, stress your body, eat up your muscle, or load you up with hidden sugars.

I don't want you to struggle anymore. Within a month, your appetite will be a healthy one and you'll crave food only when you really need nutrients; and you'll find that without your sugar addiction, you crave different types of food, perhaps for the first time in your life. You'll actually enjoy fruits, vegetables, and whole grains in a whole new way, especially because you'll have plenty of healthy fats in your diet to bring out their flavors.

The exciting thing about the Appetite Solution is that it works—regardless of your diet history, your childhood eating patterns, or your genes. In fact, eating this way transforms the way your genes express themselves, giving you the chance to push your genetic destiny into a whole new pattern.

I'll tell you exactly what I tell all of my patients: Your weight is not your fault, and neither is your appetite. All your life, you've been given the wrong information about the way your metabolism, weight, and appetite work. Maybe some of that bad information came from other books you've read. Maybe it even came from a doctor, trainer, or nutritionist. They were doing the best they could, and so were you. But nothing ever worked before—because you never had exactly the right information before.

Now you do. And the good news is that the Appetite Solution doesn't require tons of willpower, an iron discipline, or a boatload of motivation. It just takes one small step—for you to begin—and your reward for taking that step is that you never have to be hungry again.

Part I

Why Am I Always So Hungry?

Chapter 1

The Calorie Trap

I'm the classic yo-yo dieter," Angelita told me with a sigh the first time we met. A vivacious woman, Angelita carried her extra twenty pounds (9 kilos) with energy and grace, but her face was worried. "It used to be just ten extra pounds (4.5 kilos)," she told me. "Then fifteen (about 7 kilos), and now it's twenty (9 kilos). Every year, my weight is creeping up, five pounds (about 2 kilos) at a time. No matter how hard I try, I can't keep it off!"

Trying to keep her voice from trembling, Angelita described the pattern. She would start a diet and fitness program, working diligently to follow every rule of whatever diet she had adopted and to keep up with every minute of whichever exercise program she had chosen. The first week, she would lose weight—maybe even as much as five pounds (2.25 kilos), depending, as she put it, "on how much I starved myself." Still, Angelita was a disciplined, determined person, and, as she told me, "if I say I'm going to do something, I stick to it."

So Angelita endured the hunger for the first week, thrilled with her weight-loss reward. But then something seemed to freeze the scale. The second week, no weight loss. The third week, Angelita gained back two, maybe three of the pounds (between 1 and 1.5 kilos) that she had lost. And by the end of the first month on a diet-plus-weight-loss regime, she was holding steady at just two or three pounds (1 to 1.5 kilos) off her original weight—with an appetite that seemed to get more intense with every passing day.

Eventually, like most dieters, Angelita gave up. "If I was starving all the time, and I wasn't losing weight anyway, what was the point?" she asked me. "So I'd go back to eating the way I usually did—and then I'd gain five *more* pounds (2.25 kilos)." She pointed to her hips and belly, and sighed again. "And then I started gaining *ten* more pounds (2.25 kilos), and I was already ten pounds overweight—so now it's twenty (9 kilos)! Dr. Colella, how do I turn this thing around?"

I had heard Angelita's story many times before: The diet-and-exercise plans that didn't work. The weight regain that turned into weight increase. The frustration. The self-blame. The dieters who "cheated" on their exercise plans. The exercisers who cheated on their diets. The people who skimped on both, and the ones like Angelita who skimped on neither. No matter how well or badly people executed their diet-plus-exercise programs, they always seemed to end up failing.

Worst of all was the hunger. Life is too short to be miserable when you don't have to be; and Angelita, like so many people who come to me for treatment, was miserable.

"Angelita," I said to her, waiting until her eyes met mine. "This is not your fault."

I explained to her that several interlocking systems in her body are designed to hold on to every last bit of extra weight. When you cut calories—and especially when you start cutting calories and begin an exercise program at the same time—you trigger those systems. In response, they put your "fat-storing" mechanisms into overdrive.

"There is a solution," I told her. "We'll ramp up your protein intake so your body doesn't feel like it's starving.[1] Then we'll cut back very slowly on your *simple sugars*—the real culprits behind your weight gain. Two weeks later, when all that protein has assured your body that you have enough food, we'll cut back on your simple sugars more aggressively—and that's when we'll add in the exercise, too."

Angelita looked at me skeptically, unable to believe that she might have found a solution.

"We can absolutely turn this thing around," I assured her. "But first, we're going to have to do something about adaptive thermogenesis."

It's All About the Energy

As you learned in the introduction, *adaptive thermogenesis* is the process by which your body regulates its expenditure of energy.[2] Every time you eat something, you're consuming energy—measured in the form of calories. Every time you exercise, you're expending energy—which can also be measured in the form of calories.

In theory, when you want to lose weight, you can take in fewer calories by eating less, expend more calories by exercising more, or, to make a real weight-loss one-two punch, do both. That sounds good—but it's actually not the way your body works. Your body evolved from a time when food was scarce and body fat was at a premium, so it responds to "fewer calories in" and "more calories expended" in ways that often seem counterintuitive.

The first thing that happens when you cut calories is that you get hungry. Now, right there is where many people stop short. The hunger is too much for them, and they have to eat more calories to get back to what their bodies are used to.

When I meet people who tell me this story, I reassure them that this isn't their fault either. We should be glad that our body's drive to keep itself alive is so strong—even overpowering. We just have to figure out how to feed ourselves and lose weight at the same time.

But regardless of how you respond to this hunger—whether you give in to it on day one or tough it out for three months—this hunger is signaling a problem, a reason your calorie-restricted diet is doomed to fail.

Let's look at where this hunger comes from. When you restrict calories or begin a new level of exercise, your blood sugar, or *blood glucose,* level drops. Blood glucose circulates through your bloodstream to visit every single cell in your body. Glucose enters each cell thanks to the hormone insulin, and that's how your body is nourished. Your body is constructed to need a continuous supply of glucose, just as a car needs a continuous supply of gas. Glucose is your fuel; without it, your body won't function.

Your body extracts glucose from carbohydrates—grains, legumes, vegetables, fruits, and, to some extent, dairy products. Some of these carbohydrates are *complex* and some are *simple* (aka "simple sugars"), and these two types of carbs have very different effects on your blood glucose levels, your metabolism, your appetite, and your weight. But let's save that discussion for chapter 2. The main point here is that your body's cells need a steady supply of glucose in order to function, and that glucose primarily comes from carbohydrates.

When you cut calories, you cut at least some carbohydrates, and if you're on a low-carb diet, you're cutting even more. Suddenly, your body doesn't have all the glucose that it's used to. When your blood glucose levels drop from where they usually are—even if they were too high before and maybe are still too high—your body senses a reduction in the amount of energy available. Sound the alarm!

Or, more specifically, "Trigger a *stress response.*"

The Stress Mess

You might have heard that stress is bad for your weight, but perhaps you assumed that stress was a psychological phenomenon—a matter of "comfort food" or "emotional eating."

Nope. Stress is a very specific biochemical reaction that is triggered whenever your body encounters a physical or an emotional challenge—a biological reaction which virtually ensures that your body will gain or retain weight. That's why a key principle of the Appetite Solution involves short-circuiting the stress response: by loading you up with protein, not cutting your calories too quickly, not cutting your simple sugars too quickly, and delaying the point at which you begin or step up your exercise. As you will see in the rest of this chapter, all of these key strategies are designed to short-circuit the stress response and foil your wily opponent, adaptive thermogenesis.

By the way, "stress" sounds like an emotional state, but the stress response can be triggered by either a physical event or an emotional one. Pressing to meet a deadline, having an emotional call with a loved one, or staying up at night worrying about the bills can set off a stress response. So can missing a meal, cutting back on calories, or doing an unaccustomed twenty minutes on the treadmill. Whenever your body thinks that it is facing a challenge—including a possible reduction in those glucose-releasing carbs—you go into stress mode, with disastrous consequences for both your appetite and your weight.

The stress response is an intricate biological process that relies heavily on your adrenal glands, two organs located in your lower back, just above your kidneys. Your adrenals release a chemical cascade of stress hormones, including *cortisol,* one of the most powerful and misunderstood hormones in the human body. Cortisol helps shift your body's resources into emergency mode, and it's a big reason why Angelita was having trouble losing weight—and perhaps why you are, too.

One of the most troubling effects of cortisol is the way it derails your muscles. And muscles are crucial to your metabolism. So before we look at how cortisol derails your muscles, let's look at how healthy muscles function.

Muscles: Your Metabolism's Best Friend

Lean muscle mass is the best possible driver of your metabolism. A body with a high proportion of lean muscle mass burns more calories—even when it is sleeping or at rest—than a body with a low proportion of lean muscle mass. One of my ultimate goals with the Appetite Solution is to help you to enjoy a higher proportion of lean muscles, which will keep your metabolism running high and hot, burning off calories quickly and efficiently.

In fact, when you have a high enough proportion of lean muscle mass—which you can easily achieve by following the fitness plans presented in chapter 7—you will eventually achieve the metabolism of a teenager. Even if you occasionally have a piece of cake or a serving of chips, your fabulous metabolism will burn those calories off quickly because of your high proportion of lean muscle. (To be on the safe side, I'll suggest a "Protein Protocol" in chapter 11 to help you safely indulge; see page 251.)

Do you have slender friends who seem to be able to eat everything without gaining weight? If so, chances are that they have a high proportion of lean muscle mass. Their metabolism is running hotter than yours because of those muscles, so if they eat a high-calorie or high-sugar treat, they burn it off quickly instead of storing it as fat. Don't worry—by the time you finish the Appetite Solution, you'll be well on your way to a fabulous metabolism of your own.

Meanwhile, here's another thing about that lean muscle mass: It means that whenever you *do* exert yourself, your body burns hotter and expends more energy. So when your lean and muscled friends do twenty minutes on the treadmill, they are literally burning more calories than you are expending in the *same* twenty minutes—particularly if you have just started a diet or if you are not used to exercising.

That's right. Their twenty minutes on the treadmill—same pace, same time, same everything—burns more calories off that lean, muscled body than your time on the treadmill burns from yours. Their metabolism is set to burn high and hot when they are asleep, when they are at rest, and when they are exerting themselves. In all three of those situations, they are burning more energy than you are simply because of their ratio of muscle to fat.

That's how powerful muscles can be when it comes to burning calories and losing weight. And that's why, when your body thinks it's in danger of starvation, muscles are the first thing it attacks.

The Cortisol Conspiracy

So, here you are, with a low proportion of muscle relative to your body fat and a certain amount of excess fat that you would like to lose. You restrict your calories through a diet and expend some extra calories through a fitness program—which you have probably started at the same time as your diet—and during the first week, you lose three to five pounds (about 1.5 to 2 kilos).

I've already told you that this initial weight loss comes from muscle (and the water that it contains), but I haven't told you why. Now I'll give you the answer in one word: *cortisol.*

As we have just seen, your muscles burn more energy than does your fat, even when you are sleeping; and when you are physically active, your muscles burn even *more* energy. From cortisol's point of view, that is a big problem. Cortisol has just been called to the scene by a body that believes it's in danger of starvation (because of your new diet) and/or depletion (because of your new level of exercise).

So cortisol says, in effect: "Wow, those muscles are a big drain on your energy supply—a drain we can't really afford. Plus, you're taking in fewer calories all of a sudden, and we can't afford that, either. Let's kill two birds with one stone and eat up some of your muscle. That chewed-up muscle will give us some extra calories to make up for the ones you're not eating anymore. And reducing your overall muscle mass will lower your whole metabolic expenditure, leaving you with relatively less 'high-burning' muscle and relatively more 'low-burning' fat."

That's why, if you have begun your diet by cutting overall calories, or by cutting calories plus starting a fitness program, you are setting yourself up for failure. During the first two weeks of calorie restriction, cortisol facilitates the *breakdown* of muscle tissue into smaller protein molecules that are then converted to glucose, all in a desperate attempt to sustain your blood sugar levels.

This is why I tell my patients that the wrong approach to dieting is basically "eating yourself up for breakfast." If you simply cut calories and/or start a fitness program, and particularly if you do them both at the same time, that's exactly what you're going to do.

Consuming larger amounts of protein will protect your muscles and keep your body from eating them up. If you have enough protein in your system from what you eat, you don't have to get it from breaking down your own muscle tissue. I'm going to provide a plan for you that includes exactly the right amount of protein to keep your body from losing muscle mass.

But if you're on a typical restricted-calorie diet, you are often consuming less protein than usual, so you have less protein to support your all-important muscle. To make matters worse, that same cortisol-based stress response prevents your muscles from using even a regular amount of protein to repair, rebuild, and regrow. This is why the first few pounds or kilos that you lose on most diets are basically just muscle mass and water. Early fat loss simply will not happen with a restricted-calorie approach. No matter how hard you try—no matter how much you starve yourself and/or ramp up the exercise—you'll only be making things worse. Eventually, you'll get too hungry and discouraged to keep going, you'll start eating just a little bit more or exercising just a little bit less . . . and then you'll gain back the weight you lost and probably a few pounds or kilos more besides.

How Cortisol Tells Your Body to Store Fat

Let's look at yet another way that cortisol protects your body fat: via your blood sugar.

As we will see in chapter 2, when your blood sugar levels are high, your insulin levels are high also. And when your insulin levels are high, your body stores fat rather than burning it. That's why chapters 2 and 3 will focus on helping you to bring your blood sugar and insulin levels down.

Well, guess what pushes your blood sugar levels *up*? Among other things, cortisol.

Now, this gets very tricky. Normally, your blood sugar levels go *up* when you consume carbohydrates, and *down* when your level of carbs gets low.

But if you restrict calories too suddenly or in a way that your body isn't used to, your body gets stressed, triggers a cortisol release, and then cortisol pushes your blood sugar levels *up*. This is known as *gluconeogenesis,* that is, the creation of glucose, but you can think of it simply as "cortisol causing you to make more glucose."

This can happen when you miss a meal, which is why skipping meals is so bad for weight loss. But it can also happen through an overall restriction of calories—or through an unusual level of exertion in the form of exercise. It can even happen through emotional stress, such as a shakeup at work, a move to a new home, or worry about a child. Anything that stresses you, physically or emotionally, generates cortisol. And cortisol then pushes your blood sugar levels up.

Why is *that* a problem? Because when your blood sugar levels go up, so do your insulin levels. And insulin cues your body to store fat.

And cortisol doesn't simply create *high* blood sugar; it can also create *dysregulated* blood sugar, that is, blood sugar that is sometimes going up (cuing high insulin and fat storage) and sometimes dropping down fast (cuing hunger—often ravenous hunger, especially for the sweet and starchy foods that will bring your blood sugar levels back up as fast as possible). In response to either physical or emotional stress, cortisol can mess with your blood sugar in all of these ways—which in turn disrupts your appetite, your metabolism, and your weight.

Here's another way your stress hormones misguidedly attempt to help you—not cortisol, this time, but two other stress hormones known as *epinephrine* (or *adrenaline*) and *norepinephrine* (or *noradrenaline*). Your liver has stored up some extra calories to save in case you really need them. This is known as *glycogen,* and it is made from glucose. When you don't eat, epinephrine and norepinephrine stimulate *glycogenolysis,* that is, the conversion or breakdown of glycogen to glucose. They usually do this in response to the blood sugar drop that comes with fasting or missing a meal, but it can also happen with the calorie restriction or calorie burning that comes from diet and exercise.

And, as we just saw, when that glycogen becomes glucose, your blood sugar levels go up, your insulin levels also go up, and your insulin levels cue your body to store fat rather than burn it.

But we're not done yet. The stress conspiracy still has a few more ways to prevent you from losing fat.

The Stress Conspiracy

Let's go back for a bit to that fateful moment when the cortisol-induced "stress cascade" derails your efforts at weight loss and begins to destroy your muscle. Another aspect of that chemical cascade involves your thyroid gland, which creates even more obstacles to weight loss.

Your thyroid gland has many functions, but regulation of your metabolism is one of the main ones. When cortisol informs your thyroid gland that you are in imminent danger of starvation and/or depletion, that gland starts producing less thyroid hormone, which causes your metabolism to drop still farther. Now you are expending even *less* energy than you were before, which makes it even harder to lose weight.

Low thyroid hormone can make you feel tired, sluggish, depressed—and no wonder! Your body is basically trying to hibernate until you can find it some more food.[3]

The next stress conspirator is your own muscle tissue, which has its own reaction to weight loss. Your muscles want to be able to work hard for you whether you eat enough food or not. After all, since they evolved during a time when food was often scarce, they needed to be able to function even when you didn't know where your next meal was coming from.

So what happens when you start to lose weight by cutting calories? Your muscles also say, "Uh-oh, starvation!" And they find ways to work more efficiently; that is, they figure out how to burn *fewer calories with the same exertion.*[4]

If you really were starving to death, this would be a great help. Despite your scary reduction in calorie intake, your muscles would still function well enough to enable you to walk to the next village to beg some food, run from a menacing predator, or start plowing the field for the spring planting.

But if you are trying to lose twenty or thirty pounds (10 or more kilos) of excess fat, your muscles' new efficiency has just made that much, much harder. Now when you jump on the treadmill to burn off calories, your muscles are working *more* efficiently than those of your gym rat neighbor on the next treadmill, with all that lean muscle mass. You will, once again, be literally burning fewer calories from the exact same workout, because your efficient muscles have figured out how to do the same job with fewer calories.

Stress has this effect, because your body can't tell the difference between a fight with your spouse and a trek across the tundra. From your body's point of view, stress means, "We have to work harder than we're used to," and so your body responds by improving its calorie efficiency.

And—you guessed it—calorie reduction, that is, a diet, also has this effect. Your body says: "Uh-oh, less food is coming in than usual. Let's become more efficient so we can do the *same amount of work with less food.*"

And when you start a diet and a fitness program at the same time?— that's a double whammy. *More work, less food*—your muscles scramble to become as efficient as they can possibly be so that your calorie reduction and increased exertion don't let you waste away to nothing. You just want to take off a few pounds or kilos, but your body is doing its darnedest to protect against starvation and exhaustion.

Believe it or not, there is one more player in this "keep the weight on" game. And that is your autonomic nervous system.

The Last Piece of the Puzzle

The final element in adaptive thermogenesis is your *autonomic nervous system*.[5] *Autonomic* means that this is the part of your nervous system that works on its own, that is, it's automatic. Your autonomic nervous system regulates functions that we don't have conscious control over, including breathing, heart rate, blood pressure, and metabolism.

The autonomic nervous system is very flexible and adaptive. If you choose to breathe quickly and rapidly, you can; and if you choose to breathe slowly and deeply, you can usually do that, too. But if you aren't consciously thinking about it, your breathing slows down when you are at rest and speeds up when you need to pull more oxygen into your lungs—all without your telling it to do so.

This is great when it comes to basic life support, but it can make things more difficult when you are trying to lose weight. Because when the pounds or kilos come off, your autonomic nervous system says, "Uh-oh, starvation coming!" And just as it obligingly speeds up your breathing for you when you begin to run fast, it helpfully slows down your metabolism for you so you won't keep losing weight.

When you are on a calorie-restricted diet, your autonomic nervous system induces a *hypometabolic condition*—a condition of lowered metabolism—to increase your muscles' efficiency, that is, to make sure that your workout routine burns fewer calories than the identical routine of your gym rat neighbor. Your autonomic nervous system also acts to reduce your body's production of thyroid hormone, making your metabolism even more sluggish.

If you are thinking that all of this seems like a genetic and physiological conspiracy to make you fat, you are exactly right. It was a conspiracy we might have welcomed throughout most of human history, when food was scarce, exertions were urgent, and we needed every last bit of body fat to make it through the winter. Now, however, it's a conspiracy against your body's own best interests, because that extra fat is quite dangerous to your health. As we will see in chapter 2, body fat is not inert—it is metabolically active, and almost every extra ounce or gram is sending dangerous inflammatory chemicals into your body.

So yes, there is a conspiracy, with many different systems cuing your body to hold on to extra weight. It should be no surprise that the concluding words of a 2008 study published in the *American Journal of Clinical Nutrition*, "the steadily increasing prevalence of obesity in humans suggests that body fatness is facilitated more vigorously than body thinness."[6]

Appetite Solution to the Rescue

At this point, you're probably ready for some good news, so here it is: Although the stress response is quick to respond to any drop in calories or glucose, or to any increased exertion, after a week or two it begins to fatigue. At that point, your body stops eating its own muscles for breakfast. Which means that if we can just make it through those first two weeks, we can maybe get in there and make a difference.

So here's the strategy I have devised that has helped so many people— and now, you too—to lose unwanted body fat, and why, after the first two or three days, you can do it without feeling hungry:

Step One: Ramp up the protein. Extra protein is going to perform two very helpful functions to straighten up the stress mess. It will

- ☐ jam the appetite signals so hunger doesn't set off another stress response,[7] and
- ☐ protect your muscles so that your body doesn't eat them up for breakfast.[8]

Step Two: Slowly and gradually cut back on simple sugars.
Normally, when you cut back on simple sugars, you provoke a huge stress response and an enormous appetite, as your body wonders why it isn't getting its normal supply of glucose. When you wean yourself off simple sugars, you avoid the stress response, jam the hunger signals, and foil adaptive thermogenesis. We'll look at this more in the next chapter.

Step Three: After the first two weeks, begin moderate exercise.
Depending on how you're eating now, I probably won't suggest you cut many calories during your first two weeks of the Appetite Solution. You'll want to cut some simple sugars, but slowly. Still, your body will experience *some* stress just from beginning to eat in a new way. Let's give that stress response time to play itself out. After two weeks, your stress response will be fatigued, your body will have less temptation to eat its own muscle for breakfast, and you can safely begin to exercise without further damaging your muscle tissue.[9] Of course, if you are already exercising, you can keep your exercise at the same level, but don't increase it just yet.

The Exercise Bonanza

For permanent, long-term sustained weight loss, there is only one word: *exercise*. Your long-term solution lives and dies with brisk, moderate exercise, at least four times a week, a total of thirty minutes each time. This is because exercise builds muscles, increasing your ratio of muscle to fat—and that, as we saw, is what ultimately revs up your metabolism. When you follow the Appetite Solution, you can achieve the metabolism of a teenager—but you'll need to increase your lean muscle mass to get there.

But exercise is hard, right? For many people, even the thought of it gives them a cold chill. If you are not currently an exerciser, I'm sure you have said to yourself, "If exercise is essential to losing weight, then I'm out."

So here is another piece of good news: *You won't feel that way in a few weeks.*

How do I know? Because I have seen this happen for my patients time and time again.

If you feel resistant to exercise, part of the reason why is because your body is currently full of inflammatory chemicals from excess fat and inflammatory foods—foods that you'll gradually drop when you follow the Appetite Solution. We'll look more closely at inflammation in chapter 2, but for now let me just tell you that inflammation contributes to fatigue, anxiety, depression, and brain fog. It promotes muscle aches, joint pain, headache, and indigestion. Through its effect on your brain chemicals, inflammation can even make you feel less optimistic, less self-confident, and less willing to take healthy risks. If you are suffering from all those things, no wonder you don't want to exercise!

But after just two weeks of the Appetite Solution, a great deal of your inflammation will be gone (with more to go in following weeks). You'll feel stronger, clearer, and more energized. Your brain fog will have melted away. Depression will lift and anxiety will subside. The idea of moving vigorously will not feel nearly as daunting.

Then there are the motivating efforts of exercise itself. If you can stick with an activity for longer than fifteen minutes, your brain begins to release *endorphins,* those natural feel-good chemicals that promote a sense of calm and well-being. Moderate exercise has been shown to be even more effective than antidepressants in combating mild and moderate (nonclinical) depression.[10] Exercise relieves anxiety, lowers inflammation, boosts your immune system, and quite apart from any calorie expenditure, generally cues your body chemistry toward the promotion of a metabolism that burns fat rather than stores it.[11]

Moderate exercise lowers the stress response, which, as we have seen, is a prime culprit in the body's conspiracy to hold on to fat. In addition, exercise promotes healthy sleep—and sleep deprivation is another major stressor as well as an appetite inflator, as we will see in chapter 4.

In a number of different ways, including its effect on the stress response, exercise helps to stabilize your blood sugar. In chapter 2, we'll see how fluctuating blood sugar levels inflate your appetite. Here I'll just say that exercise is so good at stabilizing your blood sugar that people who are prediabetic or even actually suffering from Type II diabetes can reduce or even eliminate their need for insulin by exercising. Since insulin promotes fat storage, this is good news on the weight-loss front as well.

Recent research has unearthed yet another significant benefit of exercise. A study revealed that mice that exerted themselves secreted a hormone while they were exercising that actually reprogrammed their fat cells. Exercise, it seems, raised the mice's resting metabolism—the amount of calories burned during rest or sleep. As we have seen, lean muscle mass boosts resting metabolism as well, giving exercise at least two types of metabolic support: indirectly, through building muscle, and directly, through altering fat cells.

The hormone that effects this welcome transformation is known as *irisin,* which is released from skeletal muscle.[12] After you've come to rest, irisin may play a role in transforming your fat cells from white fat cells to brown fat cells. White fat tends to promote inflammation, whereas brown fat boosts your metabolism, so it is a far preferable type of fat to have.[13] Irisin also seems to be part of the reason that exercise stabilizes blood sugar and lowers LDL, or "bad," cholesterol levels.

Exercise also has terrific benefits for blood pressure and heart health, with a long-term reduction in the risk for heart attack and stroke. And exercise promotes joint health and helps prevent osteoporosis and osteopenia. In other words, your bones will be stronger while your whole body will be more flexible.

In your weight-loss journey, exercise is going to become your best friend as it boosts your mood, replenishes your energy, reduces your appetite, and helps you achieve the metabolism of a teenager. So if you don't feel like exercising right now, don't worry. Breathe deep, get started on Phase 1 of the Appetite Solution, and trust that your body will be in a very different place in just two weeks.

Chapter 2

The Metabolism Mystery

Let me introduce you to two hypothetical women. Both are the same age—anywhere from the teenage years into their seventies. One, let's call her Emma, has always been slender. The other, whom we'll call Meredith, is thirty pounds (13.6 kilos) heavier than her healthy weight.

Emma is only ever pleasantly hungry, right around the time for her meal or snack. The food she eats leaves her feeling full and satisfied. Sometimes she looks forward to her next meal, but usually, when she's not actually eating or cooking, she rarely thinks about food.

Meredith feels as though she thinks about food all the time. She often finds herself hungry an hour or so after she eats, and it's that ravenous, insistent hunger that makes it hard to think about anything else. Whereas Emma enjoys her hunger, Meredith feels like a prisoner of hers.

Emma usually feels clearheaded, calm, and optimistic. She feels as though she has the energy she needs to get things done. Most of the time, she sleeps well each night and wakes up refreshed. She rarely gets sick.

Meredith, by contrast, often feels foggy, anxious, and discouraged. She feels fatigued or low-energy. Sometimes she has trouble falling asleep at night. Sometimes she wakes up in the middle of the night and can't get back to sleep. She gets colds or catches a "bug" if it's going around.

Now let's look at each woman's daily diet and see whether you can figure out what's behind the metabolic differences that are affecting their appetite, mood, and health.

What Emma Eats	What Meredith Eats
Breakfast	
Porridge with fresh bananas	Porridge with raisins
Almond milk	Skimmed milk
One whole orange	Orange juice
Morning snack	
Coffee with almond milk	Coffee with fat-free coffee creamer
Wholemeal toast with peanut butter	Cinnamon bagel with "all-natural" apple butter
Plain fat-free Greek yogurt with fresh berries	Flavored fat-free strawberry yogurt
Lunch	
Grilled salmon and salad with vinegar and oil	Grilled salmon and salad with fat-free dressing
Afternoon snack	
Rice crackers and hummus	Power bar
Sliced tomato	Glass of vegetable juice
Dinner	
Grilled chicken with mango salsa	Grilled chicken with barbecue sauce
Brown rice	White rice
Steamed broccoli	Steamed broccoli
Fresh sliced apple lightly sautéed with ginger, cinnamon, and artificial sweetener	Organic applesauce

Both women eat porridge, bread, and rice. Neither woman eats sweets, baked goods, snack foods, or fried foods. You can see that both women are working hard to make healthy choices. Yet Emma's diet is geared toward metabolic success, while Meredith's diet is setting her up for metabolic failure.

Why?

From Metabolic Failure to Metabolic Success

In many ways, the two women's diets look very similar. Yet Emma's weight remains at a healthy level, her hunger is pleasant and mild, she doesn't feel like eating more food than her body needs, and she is satisfied by what she eats. Her metabolism leaves her in a calm and optimistic mood with plenty of energy for her daily tasks and lots of good support for her immune system. That is the definition of *metabolic success.*

Meredith, by contrast, is carrying excess weight and she's hungry much of the time. She often feels like eating more food than her body needs. Sometimes she resists that hunger, and sometimes she doesn't, but she is almost always struggling with her appetite. Her metabolism leaves her fatigued, mildly depressed, unable to sleep well, and with a weakened immune system. These are all signs that Meredith is suffering from *metabolic failure.*

So here's the first message I want to share with you: *Your weight is supposed to effortlessly remain at a healthy level, and your appetite is supposed to support a healthy weight. All of this happens when you achieve the correct calorie mix, with primarily 30 percent of your daily intake as lean protein.*[14] If you are carrying extra weight—whether it's five pounds, fifteen, or fifty (2, 10 or 20-odd kilos)—something is out of balance with your metabolism. And if you feel hungry for more food than you need, that's part of the same metabolic imbalance.

Likewise, if your metabolism is in balance, you are likely to have plenty of energy, a clear head, a balanced mood, and a strong immune system. An imbalanced metabolism affects your energy, brain function, mood, and immune system as well as your appetite and weight.

As I tell my patients, none of this is your fault. This is *not* about a weak will, a lack of discipline, or an emotional attachment to food. It's about eating the foods that disrupt your body's metabolism—often without even realizing that you're doing so.

If you're eating the kinds of foods that can send you into metabolic failure, your weight might be creeping slowly upward over the years, or it might simply climb to a certain level and stay there. Perhaps a stressful event triggered a weight gain—a move, a breakup, a crisis at work. Perhaps your weight gain came in response to the biological changes associated with aging or, for women, with having a baby. Maybe your weight gain has been due to some combination of these factors.

You might have tried, once or many times, to fix the problem through diet, exercise, or both. But as we just saw in chapter 1, cutting calories and starting a fitness program are often apt to trigger your nemesis, adaptive thermogenesis, particularly if you begin your diet and exercise program at the same time. You try and try, but nothing works, and the metabolic failure continues.

Whether your weight gain was slow or sudden, whether your excess weight is five pounds or fifty (2 kilos or 20-odd), whether you are a "good" dieter who follows the rules or a "bad" dieter who "cheats," it's all the same problem:

> → As long as your weight doesn't easily remain at a healthy level, as long as your appetite doesn't feel mild and pleasant instead of ravenous and overwhelming, as long as you feel like eating more food than your body needs, you are in a state of metabolic failure.

The good news is that the Appetite Solution can set you up for metabolic success and eventually help you to achieve the metabolism of a teenager. Let's see what's going wrong for Meredith and how the Appetite Solution can help.

Unraveling the Mystery

On the surface, many things about Emma's and Meredith's diets seem similar, but one key difference explains the gap between Meredith's metabolic failure and Emma's metabolic success. Meredith's diet is full of *simple sugars,* and Emma's diet focuses on *complex carbohydrates.*

Emma's Complex Carbohydrates	Meredith's Simple Sugars
Fresh bananas	Raisins
Almond milk	Skimmed milk
One whole orange	Orange juice
Almond milk	Fat-free coffee creamer
Wholemeal toast	Cinnamon bagel
Peanut butter	"All-natural" apple butter
Plain fat-free Greek yogurt with fresh berries	Flavored fat-free strawberry yogurt
Vinegar and oil	Fat-free dressing
Rice crackers and hummus	Power bar
Sliced tomato	Glass of vegetable juice
Mango salsa	Barbecue sauce
Brown rice	White rice
Fresh sliced apple lightly sautéed	Organic applesauce

So what's the difference? Why does skimmed milk disrupt your metabolism, while almond milk calms your hunger and sets you up for healthy weight loss? Why does white rice make you feel ravenous, while brown rice keeps you satisfied for several hours? What's the difference between a whole orange and a glass of juice, and why is that difference so crucial to your metabolism?

Okay, here comes the science lesson! Stay with me, because once you understand this crucial concept, you are going to feel empowered about food in a whole new way.

Simple Sugars Versus Complex Carbs

Basically, all simple sugars are carbohydrates: a combination of carbon, hydrogen, and oxygen. A simple sugar is a short chain of these molecules. A complex carbohydrate is a longer chain of these molecules, branched or twisted into a more complicated shape. In the foods where they appear, complex carbs are often interwoven with *fiber*, a tough, sturdy, and indigestible element found in grains, legumes, vegetables, and fruits.

Simple Sugars and Complex Carbs	
Simple Sugars	**Complex Carbs**
White potato	Sweet potato
White rice	Brown rice
White flour/white bread	Whole-grain flour/whole-grain bread
Corn	Beans
Cow's milk	Almond milk
Juices	Whole fruits and vegetables
Sauces	Whole fruits and vegetables
Baked or boiled fruits or vegetables	Raw, grilled, steamed, or lightly sautéed foods
Most processed foods	Most whole fruits, vegetables, grains, and legumes

Technically, we can talk about "simple sugars" and "complex sugars," or we can say "simple carbs" and "complex carbs." All carbohydrates are made of sugars; the only difference is whether their construction is *simple* or *complex*. This seemingly small distinction, however, makes a world of difference to the way your body digests, absorbs, and metabolizes each food.

Simple Sugars Go Down Easy

When you consume a simple sugar—whether it's a spoonful of granulated sugar, a bite of cake, some white potatoes, or a glass of freshly squeezed orange juice—you digest it very quickly. Because a simple sugar has no fiber—only easy-to-digest short chains—it passes quickly through your stomach into your small intestine, which absorbs it quickly, without much effort.

In fact, simple sugars are so easy to digest that your intestine has to do very little work. As a result, simple sugars are absorbed right at the top of your small intestine, the "sweet spot" where foods pass most quickly through the intestinal wall and into your bloodstream. There they contribute to rapidly elevating your blood glucose levels.

As we've seen, your blood carries glucose to every cell in your body. That's good, because your cells need to be fed almost constantly with a steady stream of glucose—especially your brain cells, which get even hungrier than the rest of your anatomy. That's why you often feel dizzy, anxious, or foggy when you haven't eaten in a while or when you're having a "sugar crash." Those symptoms tell you that your blood sugar levels are low—or, as we'll see later on, lower than what your brain and body are used to.

When you feel like you're "starving," you often crave not just any food, but specifically, simple sugars. That's because your body knows that these sugars will pass through your stomach, into your small intestine, and out into your bloodstream much faster than any other type of food.

Once your blood is full of glucose, how does that glucose get into your cells? This important function is facilitated by insulin, which is manufactured by your pancreas. The presence of high levels of blood sugar stimulates your pancreas to release a flood of insulin, which then starts the move of glucose from your bloodstream into each one of your cells.

In a healthy body, this process happens smoothly and easily every three to four hours. You consume something, perhaps a simple sugar, and it passes through your stomach and small intestine into your bloodstream. Your pancreas is alerted, and it releases insulin to usher the glucose into your cells. When most of the glucose has been moved into the cells, insulin levels subside. At that point, your blood sugar levels are lower, so you feel hungry again. You eat something else, and the whole process starts over.

The good thing about simple sugars is that they hit your bloodstream quickly, satisfying your hunger and feeding your brain and body soon after you consume them. This is even more true when you consume your sugars in liquid form, such as in a fizzy drink, juice, or sauce. Liquid sugars pass right from your stomach to your small intestine, where they sail through the efficient "sweet spot" in your intestine to reach your bloodstream within minutes.

The good thing is also a bad thing, however, if you look at what happens to your blood sugar levels and your insulin. When you consume a simple sugar, a lot of glucose hits your bloodstream at once—*bam!* This sugar shock jolts your pancreas into action, and then a lot of insulin hits your bloodstream at once—*bam bam!*

That first hit is your "sugar rush"—that feeling of being wired, excited, and "buzzed." The second hit is your "sugar crash"—that feeling of being foggy, tired, and perhaps somewhat depressed as the excess insulin quickly moves the sugar out of your bloodstream and into your cells. Of course, the sugar crash makes you crave another hit, and there you go: spinning around on the sugar cycle and well on your way to becoming a sugar addict.

Complex Carbs Take Time to Digest

Now let's look at what happens when you consume a complex carb instead of a simple one. Picture the complex carb as a kind of honeycomb, with multiple chambers holding little pockets of simple sugars. The "chambers" are the fiber—the tough element mixed in with the simple sugars to make a complex package. In order for your body to get the benefit of those sugars, that sturdy fibrous packaging has to be broken down.[15]

So first, the complex carb—the sweet potato, brown rice, or quinoa—travels much more slowly through your stomach than the simple sugar did.[16] Your stomach has to work harder at breaking down this food into a form that can pass on into the small intestine.

Then, when the complex carb finally reaches your small intestine, the simple sugars are still partially wrapped up in their fibrous honeycomb. Slowly, very slowly, your intestine starts to break apart the fibrous package, and slowly, very slowly, the simple sugars begin to be released.

As this process is happening, the complex carb is passing slowly from the top of your small intestine, where sugars pass quickly and efficiently into your bloodstream, down to the lower section of your small intestine, where absorption happens much less efficiently. The few simple sugars released when this carb was near the "sweet spot" at the top of your small intestine do hit your bloodstream relatively soon.

However, only a few simple sugars are available at that point. Many more are still wrapped up in their fibrous package as it drifts down through your intestine. And the lower in your intestine we go—the farther away from the "sweet spot"—the less efficiently sugars are passed into the bloodstream.

In addition, even when the simple sugars *are* released from the fibrous complex carb, they are often tangled up in longer chains and need to be untangled and broken apart. That also takes time, further slowing their release.

Like a time-release pill, the complex carb sends out its simple sugars slowly and gradually, as your intestine works to break apart the fiber and release the sugars. In fact, your body has to work so hard at digesting complex carbs, you actually burn some calories while doing it!

Simple Sugars Are Fast, Complex Carbs Are Slow

→ Simple sugars sail right through your stomach and small intestine, hit the "sweet spot" at the top of your intestine, and pass into your bloodstream quickly and all at once.

→ Complex carbs take much longer for your stomach and small intestine to process because of their tough, fibrous packaging. As a result, they pass into your bloodstream slowly and gradually, over time.

The Packaging Makes All the Difference

Because of the way they are digested, simple sugars add a lot of sugar to your bloodstream at once, whereas complex carbs take time to digest and thus release their sugars slowly. This explains why the same food can be *either* a simple sugar *or* a complex carb, depending on how it is processed or prepared.

Complex Carb	Simple Sugar
Fruits and vegetables	
Whole blueberry	Blueberry blenderized into your protein shake
Whole apple	Apple cooked down into applesauce
Whole orange	Juice squeezed from that orange
Raw, grilled, or sautéed tomato	Tomato cooked down into sauce
Raw, grilled, or sautéed veggies	Vegetables made into juice
Grains	
Whole wheat	Wheat processed into white flour
Brown rice	Rice with the bran removed to make it white rice

In all of these cases, the original whole food contains its sugars in a complex packaging that includes lots of fiber to slow your digestion down and make your body work harder. As a result, the sugar in a blueberry or orange is released slowly. By contrast, the blended blueberry or juiced orange is basically all sugar liberated from the fiber. It hits the sweet spot in your small intestine and goes straight through to your bloodstream.

A patient of mine recently told me about buying a salad at a health-food store. The labels on many of the seemingly healthy salads indicated that they had many grams of sugar—yet the salads contained only fresh, raw vegetables and maybe some whole grains, such as quinoa. She couldn't understand where all the sugars were coming from.

This was a case of misleading labeling. Yes, kale, cucumbers, broccoli, and other green vegetables contain sugars. But they are *complex sugars*— what I am calling complex carbohydrates. If my patient ate any of the health-food salads, the sugars in those vegetables and whole grains would be liberated slowly. Her body would work hard to digest those foods, and most of the sugars would miss the "sweet spot." Some of the tangled sugars from those complex carbs would not make it into her bloodstream at all; instead, they would pass right into her bowel and be expelled as waste.

By contrast, if she poured those exact same salad ingredients into a blender and made a supposedly healthy green juice, my patient would be drinking essentially pure sugar.[17] That's because the blending process liberates the sugars from their fibrous packaging, basically doing the work of digestion and allowing them to pass through her stomach and into her small intestine, where they would hit her sweet spot and be transported right into her bloodstream.

If she eats raw, fresh vegetables, my patient gets a slow, steady release of sugars—a healthy way to be nourished.[18] If she drinks a green juice, she gets a sudden hit of sugars—a far less healthy option, and one that could even cause her blood sugar levels to spike. As we will see, disruption of blood sugar, through spikes and by other means, is one of the factors that sets us up for metabolic failure.

How the Sugar Cycle Keeps You Hungry

There are basically three ways you end up feeling hungry:

1. **Healthy Hunger: a gradual drop in your blood sugar.** When your metabolism is working perfectly, you consume some carbohydrates, you digest them at an appropriate rate, the sugar hits your bloodstream, some insulin is released, and the sugar is gradually moved into your cells. The whole thing takes about three or four hours, leaving you pleasantly hungry for your next meal at about that time.

2. **Spikes and Crashes: when your blood sugar plummets quickly.** When your blood sugar falls too fast, you get hungry—even if your blood sugar level doesn't end up at a particularly low point. The rate of falling itself cues your body that something is wrong. That's why eating a simple sugar, especially without some protein to accompany it, can trigger a feeling of hunger even when you're "full." The fast infusion of sugar causes your blood sugar to spike, and then the quick flood of insulin it provokes causes your blood sugar to fall much more quickly than your body expects. That fast drop—regardless of the total amount of your blood sugar—provokes hunger.

3. **High, Unstable Blood Sugar: when your blood sugar is chronically too high, and then it drops, even slightly.** This happened recently to Janelle, one of my patients. She used to eat sweet rolls and muffins for breakfast, but when she wanted to lose weight, she switched to a plain bagel and a glass of fresh orange juice. Unbeknownst to Janelle, the bagel and orange juice were loaded with sugar—but they had somewhat *less* sugar than a sweet roll or muffin. So although Janelle's blood sugar levels were still persistently elevated, they were slightly lower than her body was used to. This was enough to trigger a "starvation" message that kept her hungry all morning long.

As you can see, when you enjoy metabolic success, you are hungry only when your body really needs more food, that is, when your cells need more glucose and there isn't enough sugar in your blood to feed them. In this state of healthy hunger, you

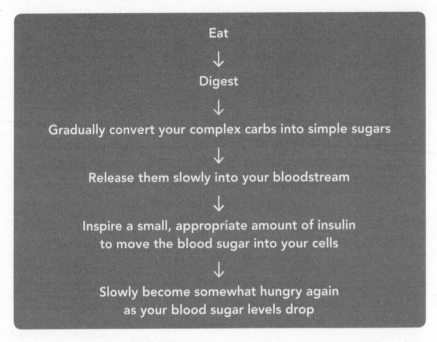

In the second two conditions I described, however, you get hungry long *before* your body actually needs more food. This is a state of metabolic failure, that is, when you are feeling hungry because your blood sugar levels are falling rapidly, or because they are somewhat lower than the unhealthy high levels that you have become used to.

This state of metabolic failure is what turns your appetite into a relentless enemy, always on the prowl for more food—and especially for those seductive simple sugars that can push your blood sugar back up quickly. Your hunger might be the constant, nagging kind, when you never feel really satisfied, or that overwhelming, devastating kind, when it feels like you're going to die if you don't eat. Either type of hunger is your clue that your metabolism is failing you.

This can feel like an emotional problem or a lack of willpower, but I promise you, it's not—it's a *biological* problem. Your blood sugar and insulin response are simply not working the way nature intended. As a result, you are always thinking about your next meal, or craving foods you try to resist, or feeling ravenous soon after you've eaten. That's not your fault; that's what happens when your metabolism is failing you. The Appetite Solution will help you turn metabolic failure into metabolic success.

Why Doesn't My Blood Sugar Level Test as "High"?

When I explained the three types of hunger to Janelle, she was with me for a while. But then she stopped and shook her head.

"Wait a minute," she said. "You're telling me that my blood sugar has been too high, and that even though it's now slightly lower, it's still too high. But I've had my blood sugar tested by my regular doctor, and she told me it was fine, not high!"

This is a common problem with the way medicine handles blood sugar readings. A lab test called hemoglobin A1c measures your average blood sugar levels over the past three months. Those levels are compared with a range that is generalized from the "average" blood sugar levels of the "average" person.

If you score too high outside this range, we consider that you have diabetes—a level of blood sugar that is so high, it tells us that your body is not making enough insulin to effectively move the blood sugar into your cells. But if you score in the "Goldilocks" middle region—neither too high nor too low, but "just right"—then we assume that you have a healthy level of blood sugar.

Unfortunately, this system is a very blunt instrument. You can easily score in the "normal" range and be heading toward developing diabetes. You can also score in the "normal" range and have blood sugar levels that are *too high for your own body.* Certainly, you can score in the "normal" range and have blood sugar levels that are higher than they were a year ago—but are still considered "normal" by most doctors.

However, I'm not happy when any of my patients has blood sugar readings in the high-normal range. I'm even less happy when the patients who have those readings are also overweight, because I know there's a connection. I know that the factors that are driving up their blood sugar levels— even when those levels may be considered "normal"—can also be the factors that make it so hard for them to lose weight. And if an overweight patient tells me that he or she is also hungry most of the time, I know that the high blood sugar levels are part of that problem, too—even if, based on routine medical practice, those readings would still be considered "normal."

So if you are more than ten pounds (4.5 kilos) overweight, I promise you, even if your tests are interpreted as "normal" by your regular doctor, your blood sugar levels could be too high for your individual body. If they weren't, you might have temporarily gained ten pounds (4.5 kilos), but you would have immediately lost it, without even trying, as your successful metabolism corrected the temporary error.

Here's the other way I know that high blood sugar levels are linked to your excess weight. Insulin, cued by that excess blood sugar, is flooding your body at higher and higher levels. You might be getting too much insulin at one time—such as after a big meal full of simple sugars or perhaps after a large, sweet dessert. Or you might be getting too much insulin throughout the day, as you continue to consume small but steady amounts of simple sugars. Either way, that excess insulin isn't just moving the blood sugar into your cells, it's also cuing your body to *gain weight*.

The Insulin Insult:
How Excess Insulin Cues Your Body to Store Fat

Now we're at the place where the rubber meets the road—where the weight gain and fat storage actually happen. What happens when you consume too many simple sugars?

The first thing is that a whole bunch of glucose hits your bloodstream, provoking a rush of insulin. The insulin moves all the glucose it can into your cells—but because you ate more simple sugars than your body needs or can use, some sugar is left over. Where does it go?

Basically, your insulin has three choices here—and only one of them is even mildly good. The first choice is to convert some of the glucose to *glycogen,* which is stored in the liver. Glycogen is basically a "sugar storage" facility. If you skip a meal, your liver converts some glycogen to glucose so that you don't literally starve to death while waiting for the next time you can eat.

After your "glycogen warehouse" is full, however, your insulin has only two choices left: convert your excess glucose to body fat, or convert it into *lipids,* that is, blood fats. These lipids take the form of cholesterol and triglycerides, which is why losing weight often brings a drop in cholesterol and why the Appetite Solution will almost certainly have that effect.

Although for years we were told that excess consumption of saturated fat results in high levels of cholesterol, we now understand that excess consumption of *sugar* also has this effect. You may not have heard this from your doctor, but I assure you, it's true. When you eat more sugars in one sitting than your body can absorb, insulin ensures that they become either body fat (weight gain) or blood fats (cholesterol and triglycerides).

Note that I didn't say, "when you consume too much sugar over the course of a week," or even a day. While eating too much sugar over time is probably the worst thing you can do if you are already experiencing metabolic failure, even consuming too much sugar *in one meal* can produce an immediate bump in the weight-gain process. When you are in your current state of metabolic failure, your insulin literally has nowhere else to put the excess sugar.

Down the road, after you have embraced the Appetite Solution and are enjoying the successful metabolism of a teenager, your body will have a different choice. By that point, you will have built up enough lean muscle mass that your sugar-burning capacity will be greatly increased. If you eat a little extra at that point, your metabolism can generally burn it off, as long as you don't overdo it. (I'll give you exact guidelines in chapter 11.)

At this point, though, when you are still overweight, your insulin response guarantees that excess sugar consumption will result in either fat storage, high cholesterol readings, or both. That's why I want you to cut back on simple sugars.

Of course, you can get the same problematic result from eating too many complex carbohydrates. With too many complex carbs, you can also end up with high blood sugar levels and an insulin response that converts sugar into fat. But it is actually not so easy to overeat complex carbs; all that fiber slows you down and makes you feel full.[19] And when you are eating the amounts of protein I recommend, overdoing the complex carbs becomes even more difficult because the protein blunts your hunger. That's why I start you off with the protein push and *then* have you cut back on the carbs, both simple and complex—slowly and gradually, so you don't even miss them. And you can still consume quite a decent amount of complex carbs, as long as you cut back on simple sugars.

Remember, another key problem with excess consumption of simple sugars is that it gives you persistently high blood sugar levels—higher than is really healthy. Those persistently high blood sugar levels in turn trigger persistently high insulin levels—and that insulin is continually telling your metabolism to store fat. In other words, blood sugar isn't just a onetime problem of spike and crash; it's also a cumulative problem that gets worse and worse the more sugars you consume throughout the day.

Perhaps at this point you are wondering why you can't simply cut calories to lose weight, especially if your calorie-cutting takes the form of carb-cutting. In theory, a low-carb diet *would* help you lose weight, but as we saw in chapter 1, it doesn't actually work that way in practice. That's because cutting calories, especially carbs, sets off a stress response and triggers adaptive thermogenesis.

So here's your takeaway:

> → If you consume too many simple sugars in a single meal, or too many simple sugars over the course of a day, your blood sugar will be persistently elevated to an unhealthy level. This spurs your insulin to convert that excess sugar into body fat, cholesterol, or both.

The Magic Rule of 5 and 20

- ☐ Don't eat more than 5 grams of simple sugars at one meal or snack.
- ☐ Don't eat more than 20 grams of simple sugars in one day.

Note that I say *simple* sugars. You'll find them in processed and refined foods, juices, sauces, and cow's milk, and, of course, in foods sweetened with sugar, honey, agave, maple syrup, all-natural fruit juices, and other similar sweeteners. Don't count the sugars in whole fruit, vegetables, grains, and legumes because they are *complex* sugars. Only *simple* sugars count toward your total.

Of course, during the first six weeks of the Appetite Solution, you don't have to count sugars at all, because I've done it for you in your meal plans for Phases 1, 2, and 3 (see chapter 5). Going forward, however, you'll want to follow this Magic Rule, with rare exceptions that I explain in chapter 10.

The Inflammation Factor

Simple sugars play havoc with your body in another way: they cause *in-flammation*.[20] Inflammation is a complex immune-system response that occurs whenever your body feels under attack. Your immune system brings out its killer chemicals to zap any invader that might threaten your safety. Unfortunately, those killer chemicals can do a lot of harm to your body as well.

Inflammation is not a problem when it's *acute,* that is, when it's a one-time response to, say, a virus or bacteria. But when inflammation is *chronic,* that is, when it basically just hangs around in your system all the time because your body keeps feeling as though something's wrong, you get all sorts of dire health problems, including weight gain.

One of the major sources of inflammation is—you guessed it—simple sugar. If you can lower your blood sugar levels and keep yourself from eating large quantities of sugar at one sitting or in one day, you can bring down your inflammation levels almost immediately. Follow the Magic Rule of 5 and 20—at most 5 grams of simple sugars at any one time and at most 20 grams over the course of a day—and you will be fighting inflammation as well as losing weight.

Inflammation creates a truly vicious cycle because as we saw in the previous chapter, fat cells themselves—especially the belly fat that simple sugars often provoke—are also inflammatory.[21] Basically, your excess weight adds to your inflammation, which in turn promotes more weight gain.

Here's another reason not to kick off your diet by cutting calories: If you simply restrict your food intake, your body perceives it as stress—and stress is an inflammatory trigger. You're far better off easing into a new way of eating and ramping up the protein before cutting back too heavily on the calories. That's a no-stress approach that your body, and your weight, will appreciate.

The Inflammation/Appetite Scale of Foods

Guess what? The very same foods that provoke inflammation also stimulate your appetite. But you can turn that vicious cycle into a "virtuous" cycle by avoiding simple sugars and other inflammatory foods. By doing so, you will

☐ bring down the inflammation that is attacking your organs from within and putting you at risk for numerous medical problems, including heart disease, autoimmune conditions, and cancer;
☐ keep inflammation from cuing your body to gain weight; and
☐ keep insulin from flooding your body, provoking an excessive appetite.

Ultimately, the Appetite Solution is also the Inflammation Solution. So here is the Inflammation/Appetite Scale of Foods, starting with the most inflammatory and ending with your healthiest choices. By following the Appetite Solution, you will eventually avoid foods numbered 6 to 10, eat moderate amounts of foods numbered 5, and enjoy the healthy benefits of foods numbered 1 to 4.

10. **Liquids that primarily consist of simple carbohydrates (sugar):** fruit juice, regular fizzy or soft drinks (sweetened with sugar), alcohol, flavored coffee drinks, sugar-sweetened tea (including anything sweetened with honey), energy drinks made with sugar (including most workout drinks), milkshakes, ice cream, and sugar-sweetened gelatin. Also boiled sweets, cough drops, and chewing gum sweetened with sugar.

9. **Pureed or thickened foods made with large amounts of sugar:** applesauce, sugar-sweetened yogurt, light or fat-free yogurt made with high-fructose corn syrup, sugar-sweetened desserts or sugar-free desserts made with high-fructose corn syrup, canned or processed fruit, baby food, mashed potatoes, cream pies, flavored syrups or toppings, dips, and sugar-free syrups made with high-fructose corn syrup.

8. **"Sweets,"** such as candy bars, cakes, and pies.

7. **Fried carbohydrates and unhealthy "fatty" foods,** such as hot dogs, chips, doughnuts, most margarine and shortening, and many processed frozen foods.

6. **More solid foods made with large amounts of simple carbohydrates (sugar):** most breakfast cereals (watch out for "other carbohydrates" listed on the label), porridge with brown sugar, white bread (it is the equivalent of having dessert during dinner), pasta, baked potatoes, biscuits, crackers, crisps, processed snack foods, pretzels, cream-based soups, and nachos with cheese (a double whammy!).

5. **Whole-grain bread and whole-grain pasta.**

4. **Complex carbohydrates, that is, vegetables and fruits.** The brighter the color, the better.

3. **Lentils and soy protein:** Lentils, soybeans, and tofu, most of which are great sources of lean protein and also contain complex carbohydrates.

2. **Healthy sources of protein and fat:** most cuts of red meat, eggs, unsweetened peanut butter (in moderation), and a variety of nuts such as almonds and walnuts.

1. **Healthy sources of lean protein:** skinless chicken breast, most white fish (no breading, and don't even think about frying it!), tuna, scallops, prawns, most cuts of pork, salmon (smoked salmon is a ready-made, easy-access, perfect source of protein), and very-low-sugar protein shakes.

We saw in the last chapter that protein supports your muscles, which boosts your metabolism, and we'll see in the next chapter that protein can jam the hunger signal, which calms your appetite.

What Else Makes You Hungry? Cutting the Gordian Knot

Simple sugars aren't the only factor making you hungry. Many other factors can have that effect, challenging your metabolism and also triggering inflammation. In fact, sometimes it seems to me that just about everything involved in modern life conspires to make us hungry! Here are just a few of the reasons that you can end up feeling hungrier than normal, with a particular craving for simple sugars:

- ☐ **Missing meals.** Nothing spins you into a sugar cycle faster than missing a meal. I've had many patients brag to me about forgetting to eat or even deliberately skipping a meal as a way of restricting calories, and my response is always the same: "I want you eating *more* often, not less!" As we saw in the previous chapter, calorie restriction not only does not help you lose weight, it can actually make it much, much harder to do so. And skipping a meal tells your body, "Watch out, food is scarce, go into starvation mode right away!" Not only are you ravenous by the time you finally do eat, you're craving simple sugars as a source of quick energy, and your metabolism is cued to hold on to every ounce of fat in case you face "starvation" again. Eating healthy meals and snacks every three to four hours, with no more than 5 grams of sugar at a time and no more than 20 grams over the course of the day, is a much better way to produce a healthy appetite and a healthy weight.

- ☐ **Not getting enough sleep,** especially on a regular basis. Even one bad night can make you extra hungry the next day, craving bagels, pasta, or something sweet. The sugar cycle is bad enough, but without enough sleep, you get the sugar cycle on warp drive![22]

- ☐ **Stress.** This can be physical stress, like an extra-heavy workout at the gym, or emotional stress, like a fight with a loved one. Stress can cause us to crave "comfort foods." This is not just an emotional response but also a biological one. Sugars cue your body to produce endorphins, natural painkillers and "feel-good" chemicals that are also appetite stimulants.

- ☐ **Medications,** especially antibiotics, antidepressants, antianxiety medications, NSAIDs (nonsteroidal anti-inflammatory drugs, such as aspirin and ibuprofen), narcotic painkillers, and medications intended to lower your blood pressure. These medications can disrupt your biology in a wide variety of ways—all of which can have problematic consequences for your metabolism, your appetite, and your weight.

☐ **Depression.** Most people who are depressed, besides feeling a considerable amount of emotional pain, have low levels of central-nervous-system serotonin. It makes sense that you would crave sweets and simple sugars in this state, since they do seem to provide some temporary relief. Unfortunately, after the sugar rush makes you feel better, the sugar crash makes you feel worse. The inflammation caused by simple sugars, which you learned about on page 51, can also intensify your depression. The Appetite Solution, by contrast, is a natural *anti*depressant and can actually improve your mood through its reduction in simple sugar intake.

☐ **Anxiety.** Like depression, anxiety creates emotional pain and is correlated with low serotonin levels. It's not surprising that you crave simple sugars when you feel anxious, but unfortunately, spinning into the sugar cycle can actually make your anxiety intensify. Again, the Appetite Solution can bring you some relief.

☐ **Heartburn.** Gastroesophageal reflux disease (GERD), or "heartburn," occurs when the contents of your stomach backwash up into your esophagus—the "swallowing tube" that connects your throat to your stomach. Some stomach acid comes along with the food, causing a burning sensation. If you've suffered from heartburn, you might have noticed that it often sparks a desire to eat. That's because you're instinctively trying to find something that will absorb the excess acid and stop the burning. Foods high in simple sugars—including milk and starchy "white foods" (potatoes, pasta, white rice)—seem soothing and helpful in this context, even though they spin you right back into the sugar cycle. If heartburn is a problem for you, particularly if you frequently take antacids or heartburn medications, see a physician who can evaluate your condition and provide proper treatment.

To make matters even more complicated, all of these factors—and many others—interact with one another. Anxiety keeps you from sleeping. Lack of sleep makes you depressed. Missing a meal ramps up your stress. Overeating and excess weight contribute to heartburn. As Janelle found, learning about these many interactions can feel overwhelming; they seem like a tangle of restrictions that just keeps you trapped.

Luckily, in this case, the solution is far simpler than the problem. It makes me think of that old story of the Gordian knot, set in the ancient Turkish city of Gordium. According to legend, the Gordian knot could not be untied. If you pulled on one strand, it would just make the knot tighter, binding all the other strands more closely. Pull on another strand, and you'd get the same result. Attacking any one individual strand only made the knot more difficult to untie.

As legend has it, Alexander the Great rode into the city, was confronted with the knot, and whipped out his sword. Instead of trying to untangle all the individual threads, Alexander simply cut through the entire knot in one fell swoop.

That's what the Appetite Solution will do for you. *Increasing your protein intake* unsheathes the sword. *Cutting back on simple sugars* slices the knot to shreds. *Adding some moderate exercise at the beginning of Week 3* will guarantee victory over your appetite, help you return to a healthy weight, and, ultimately, give you the metabolism of a teenager. No matter how many factors are inflating your appetite, and no matter how persistently they all interact with one another, the Appetite Solution will transform your appetite and reduce your weight.

A New Teenage Metabolism

Janelle was excited about a new way of eating that would transform her appetite and enable her to drop her excess weight. To her delight, Phase 1 of the Appetite Solution did indeed leave her feeling full and satisfied after every meal. And when she finished Phase 2, she was thrilled to see that she was halfway to her goal weight. Within a few weeks more, she had reached her goal, feeling both more satisfied and more energized than she had in a long time.

Janelle was also pleased that with her new teenage metabolism, she could occasionally indulge in some of her old favorite foods, although, she said, those foods had lost a lot of their appeal. "I still like chips *once* in a while," she told me, "but I don't feel like I have to have them every day, or even a few days a week." As her appetite changed, Janelle realized how much of her previous eating had been driven by what she now saw as a sugar addiction.

"Honestly, it feels good to be done with that," she told me on her last visit. "It feels great to be slim—but it feels even better to be free!"

Chapter 3

Your Secret Sugar Saboteurs

Greg, whom we met in the introduction, eats a 2,000-calorie diet that has no grains or starches and includes lots of fresh fruits and vegetables. As we saw, he lives on protein shakes with fresh blueberries, an occasional glass of freshly squeezed orange juice, salads with grilled salmon and low-fat dressing, fat-free vanilla yogurt, and skimmed decaf lattes. He also keeps himself well hydrated with water flavored with lemon wedges. For dinner, he eats chicken or fish grilled with barbecue sauce or simmered in tomato sauce with lots of green vegetables on the side.

Greg's diet *sounds* healthy; however, he hasn't been able to lose more than two or three pounds (1 to 1.5 kilos) in three months, and he's perpetually hungry. Why?

As we saw in the introduction, the answer lies in the surprisingly high amount of simple sugars that lurk in Greg's diet: in his blended blueberries, fresh orange juice, low-fat salad dressing, and flavored yogurt, not to mention the additional sugars to be found in his lattes (skimmed milk), water (lemon juice), and grilled lean meats (tomato sauce and barbecue sauce). Even though Greg sticks diligently to his 2,000-calorie limit, his "healthy" diet actually includes 100 grams of simple sugars—far higher than the recommended 20 grams that you'll be eating when you follow the Appetite

Solution. These sneaky sugar saboteurs are inflating Greg's appetite and making it impossible for him to lose weight.

On the advice of her doctor, Patrice is following a 1,500-calorie low-fat diet. She sticks strictly to the printed instructions he gave her, but somehow the weight just isn't coming off. Patrice, too, is perpetually hungry, as well as extremely frustrated.

Patrice's downfall, of which she is completely unaware, are all the little extra sugar-bearing foods that she never thinks of as food. She'll add a dollop of ketchup to flavor her low-fat turkey burger, for example, oblivious to the fact that each tablespoon of ketchup contains 3 to 4 grams of simple sugars. Maybe she'll add a little relish, too: 4.4 grams per tablespoon. And of course, like most people, Patrice uses a few tablespoons of each.

Patrice loves coffee, which she loads up with skimmed milk—more simple sugars. For her three or four coffees a day, Patrice probably uses up to 8 ounces (240 millilitres) of skimmed milk—another 12.3 grams of simple sugars. Sometimes Patrice drops a spoonful of honey into some herbal tea—17 grams per tablespoon. Since her doctor has told her to avoid fat, Patrice doesn't butter her toast—instead, she uses apple butter (6 grams per tablespoon) or "all-natural" fruit jam (6 grams per tablespoon for the all-natural orange marmalade, 8 grams for the redcurrant jelly, 10 grams for the apricot preserve).

Something that Patrice would never even think of counting as food are her favorite cough drops, which she frequently pops when her mouth feels dry. Each cough drop, though, contains as much as 3.2 grams of simple sugar, and Patrice usually has three or four over the course of a day. By the time she goes to bed, Patrice is still hungry; her 1,500-calorie diet has turned into an unsuspected 2,800; plus she's consumed more than 70 grams of simple sugars—more than three times the recommended healthy amount.

Roxy would be shocked if you accused her of "cheating" in any area of her life, her diet included. "I don't cheat, I swap," she'd say, because whenever Roxy eats a few bites of a "forbidden food," she makes sure to cut out even more calories somewhere else.

Roxy has been trying for several months to lose weight with a 1,500-calorie Mediterranean-style diet, but she's never lost her taste for the sweet foods she grew up enjoying. So she skips the healthy 500-calorie breakfast recommended on the diet and has a 10 A.M. blueberry muffin instead.

"Blueberries are healthy, aren't they?" she says. "And the muffin is only 426 calories, so I'm 74 calories ahead." Maybe so, but that blueberry muffin has 37 grams of simple sugars, almost twice as much as the recommended daily amount of 20 grams.

Throughout the week, Roxy finds ways to make similar swaps— skipping the quinoa at dinner to have a few bites of her husband's potato gratin; passing on the cracked-whole-wheat tabouleh salad to have a little white rice from her best friend's lunch. The swaps feel even less like real food to Roxy because they are such small amounts and rarely from her own plate—but by the end of the day, she's not losing weight, she's perpetually hungry, and her system is overloaded with as many as 120 grams of simple sugars.

You must not forget "The Magic Rule of 5 and 20" (see chapter 2):

☐ Don't eat more than 5 grams of simple sugars at one meal or snack.

☐ Don't eat more than 20 grams of simple sugars in one day.

And remember that this rule is about *simple* sugars, not *complex* sugars such as those in whole fruit, vegetables, grains, and legumes. Only *simple* sugars count toward your total.

Your Sneaky Sugar Saboteurs

Greg, Patrice, and Roxy are all being sabotaged by simple sugars because they don't realize how sugar affects their appetite and how even small amounts of it can undermine every other weight-loss effort. Perhaps most insidiously, these people—like most—don't have any idea of how many places simple sugars lurk.

Most of us realize that simple sugars can be found in sweetened breakfast cereals, chocolate bars, ice cream, and cake. But barbecue sauce? Fresh-squeezed juice? Lemon-flavored water?

Simple sugars are also found in foods that have been sweetened with sugar, honey, agave, high-fructose corn syrup, rice syrup, cane sugar, or "all-natural" fruit juices. You'll find simple sugars in flavored yogurt, tomato sauce, fruit juice, and vegetable juice; in relish, ketchup, many mustards, and most fat-free dairy creamers; in soups and salad dressings, corn and potatoes, skimmed milk and many protein bars. They are in any food made with white flour. In fact, they are in just about every packaged or processed food you can buy, including the "all-natural" and "organic" ones: crisps, pretzels, salsa, ready meals, frozen dinners . . . the list goes on and on.

Simple sugars are in a thousand different places that you'd never expect. And they have a devastating effect on your health, your appetite, and your weight.

Even if you are torturing yourself to stay on a low-calorie, low-carb, low-fat diet, simple sugars can creep into your meals in the most unexpected ways: tomato sauce, skimmed milk, and the whole berries you buzz in your smoothie. And they lie in wait in some of those comfort foods that you have "just a bite of" because you've "been so good" the rest of the week.

If you are already overweight, however, even a bite or two of a high-sugar food is enough to derail your appetite and your metabolism. Simple sugars act upon your body chemistry to promote weight gain, fat storage, and worst of all, belly fat. They make you feel hungry all the time, even when you're so stuffed that you can barely eat another bite. If they do leave you satisfied for an hour or two, they soon spark up your hunger again before you've even had time to fully digest your food. The type of hunger simple sugars provoke is most often the craving for yet more sugar. And once your body is running on sugar, you are stuck in a kind of metabolic quicksand, and it's virtually impossible to lose weight.

So now I'm going to teach you how to become an expert sugar detective so that you can recognize simple sugars—and then swap them out for satisfying foods that won't have the same disastrous effects on your appetite, metabolism, and weight. Then we'll look at why ramping up your protein helps you to dissolve your sugar cravings, soothe your appetite, and shed those excess pounds or kilos.

Loading up on protein and cutting back on simple sugars is a winning combination. When you start Phase 1 of the Appetite Solution, Push the Protein, the extra protein will help to soothe your appetite. By Day 4, you won't feel anything more than a mild, pleasant hunger whenever it's time for you to eat. When the protein has had its effects, you'll be ready for Phase 2, Shelve the Sugar, where you gradually lower your sugar intake to a healthy level. In Phase 3, Shed the Fat, you'll be enjoying rapid weight loss—three to five pounds (about 1.5 to 2 kilos) per week—as you maintain your healthy high-protein and low-sugar combination.

Your ultimate goal: to achieve the metabolism of a teenager, with a pleasant appetite, a healthy weight, and the ability to indulge periodically in some of your favorite treats.

How to Skip the Sugar and Never Miss It

- ☐ Switch from high-sugar foods to satisfying low-sugar options that can be eaten in the same way, for example:
  - White potato → sweet potato
  - White rice → brown rice
  - Barbecue sauce → mango salsa (see recipe on page 260)
  - Tomato sauce → grilled or lightly sautéed fresh tomatoes (see recipe on page 258)
- ☐ Ramp up the protein
  - Jams the hunger signal
  - Helps you feel full
  - Supports your metabolism by building and sustaining lean muscle mass

High-Fructose Corn Syrup: Your Appetite Nemesis

If I could ban one food additive, it would probably be high-fructose corn syrup (HFCS). Introduced into our nation's food supply in the late 1970s and early 1980s, this sugar substitute is made from processed corn, and it's in just about every packaged or processed food you can imagine. I am not exaggerating when I say that this is easily one of the most detrimental foods the human organism has ever encountered.

You can find this tasty toxin in flavored yogurt, bread, canned soup, jam, applesauce, honey-roasted peanuts, energy bars, breakfast cereals, and your favorite condiments.

Researchers at Yale University recently shed new light on just how sneaky HFCS can be. These scientists used a special type of scan to track blood flow in the brain of twenty healthy young people of normal weight before and after they consumed beverages containing either fructose (the type of sugar found in high-fructose corn syrup) or glucose (the type of sugar found in table sugar).[23]

The scans revealed that when people drank the beverage containing glucose, the areas of their brains responsible for hunger were temporarily suppressed; that is, the glucose drink made them feel full. By contrast, when people drank beverages sweetened with fructose, their brains basically didn't respond. Although high concentrations of simple sugars had caused their blood sugar levels to spike, their brains had no idea that food had been consumed. As a result, all of these sugars had zero effect on their appetite.

So if you consume foods or beverages containing HFCS, your body will continue being hungry long after you have eaten the amount that "should" satisfy it. If you're hungry and you try to satisfy your hunger by eating something sweetened with HFCS—or with "natural" fruit juices, which also contain a lot of fructose—you'll stay hungry, and you'll gain weight.

In my view, that is a dastardly stunt. Don't let the food industry get away with it! Eliminating this toxic sweetener from your diet—permanently—is one of the single most important things you can do to soothe your appetite and achieve a healthy weight.

Eleven Other Tasty Toxins

I hope by now I've persuaded you to always check the label of every item you buy, searching for the simple sugars. You want to look in two places: for the total number of "sugars" listed under the nutritional information, and at the ingredients list itself, to see whether any sweeteners have been added.

However, sweeteners aren't always called "sugar." Here are some of the other common names for "sugar":

☐ Agave

☐ Barley malt

☐ Cane juice

☐ Dextrin and dextrose

☐ Dried fruit, including raisins

☐ Honey

☐ Malt syrup

☐ Maple syrup

☐ Molasses

☐ Natural fruit juices or fruit juice concentrate

☐ Rice syrup

Notice that supposedly "healthy" and "natural" sweeteners such as agave, honey, maple syrup, and fruit juices are on the list. Organic or "natural" foods often use these sweeteners, giving the impression that they are somehow better for you than regular old table sugar, rice syrup, or HFCS. But don't be fooled. These purportedly healthy foods are just as disastrous for your weight, metabolism, and appetite as any other type of sugary sweetener. When you are overweight, your body turns these sugars right into fat, and your appetite goes off the charts, just the same as happens with those sugars with less fancy names.

Your Seven Safe Sweet-Tooth Foods

Sugar or no sugar, I don't ever want you to feel deprived. Your thirty-day Appetite Solution will always keep you feeling full and satisfied, and by the time you're choosing your own foods, your appetite will be pleasant and mild, rather than ravenous and overwhelming. In chapter 8, I'll also give you a lot of suggestions for how to switch out foods that are high in sugar for healthier choices that feel very similar.

Meanwhile, let me reassure your nagging sweet tooth that it never needs to miss its sweet treats. Here are seven safe and healthy sweets you can easily enjoy while following the Appetite Solution, all of which have few if any grams of simple sugars:

☐ Sugar-free gelato, which you can have once a week—but check the brand, because many are full of sugars even when they are labeled "sugar-free" (see Resources)

☐ Sugar-free chocolate syrup

☐ Sugar-free strawberry syrup

☐ Sugar-free applesauce

☐ Sugar-free desserts

☐ Any type of fresh fruit—apples, bananas, mangos, pears, berries, grapes—but not blended, baked, or juiced and never in a can; sweeten them with your favorite artificial sweetener if you like.

☐ Unsweetened almond or coconut milk: make hot chocolate, mousse, or whipped cream; put it on your porridge with your favorite sugar-free sweetener; or fix yourself a foamy latte. Coconut milk is heavier, so if you're craving whipped cream or mousse, use that, adding a little artificial sweetener if you want some extra sweetness. Coconut milk also makes better lattes and cappuccinos than almond milk does.

Sugar, Sugar, Everywhere

Now it's time for you to become a sugar detective so that you can identify sugar saboteurs wherever they lurk. Finding them is often quite counterintuitive. Why should a baked white potato be a problem food, while a baked sweet potato is okay? Why should corn be a problem, while beans are fine? Why should fruit juices be a problem, while fresh fruit is a healthy choice? The answer lies not in calories, but in chemistry. So here's your tour of the top sugar hideouts.

1. White Foods

"White foods"—white potatoes, white rice, and anything made with refined white flour, such as baked goods, pancakes, and the like—don't necessarily have a lot of simple sugars. But they do contain a lot of starch that converts very quickly to simple sugar as soon as it hits your digestive tract.

Just as a blended blueberry or a juiced orange has had its fiber stripped away from its simple sugars, so a white food has had its fiber and other elements stripped away from its starches. In effect, both types of food have been "predigested" so that instead of taking a nice long time to digest while releasing their sugars slowly, they release their sugars almost as soon as they make it through your stomach. Just like high-sugar foods, white foods are quickly absorbed into your bloodstream, where they play havoc with your metabolism, your appetite, and your weight. Even though they are not technically high in simple sugars, they behave in the same way. So stay away from white foods.

Sugar Saboteurs

☐ White potatoes in any form: baked or boiled, but especially mashed, fried, or in a soup

☐ White bread, that is, bread made from refined flour

☐ Baked goods made with white flour: cake, biscuits, muffins

☐ Pancakes, waffles, and crepes made with refined flour

☐ White rice, that is, rice that has been refined

Appetite-Friendly Alternatives

☐ Sweet potatoes: baked, steamed, or sautéed

☐ Whole-grain breads

☐ Brown rice

☐ Quinoa

☐ Cracked bulgur wheat

☐ Buckwheat

☐ Almond flour

2. Corn and Corn Products

Think of how sweet a nice fresh ear of corn on the cob tastes, and you'll realize instantly how much sugar this grain contains: 5.6 grams in one large ear of corn. When you have the metabolism of a teenager, you might be able to indulge occasionally, but for now, say no to corn.

Sugar Saboteurs

- ☐ Corn in any form: fresh, frozen, canned, creamed
- ☐ Corn chips
- ☐ Tortillas
- ☐ Corn bread
- ☐ High-fructose corn syrup (see above)

Appetite-Friendly Alternatives

- ☐ Beans: black, red, white, navy, pinto
- ☐ Chickpeas/garbanzo beans
- ☐ Rice crackers
- ☐ Wholemeal pita bread
- ☐ Baked goods made with no sweeteners and with whole-grain flour or almond flour

3. Condiments

One of my most successful patients tells a story of how, once she had cut all the other simple sugars out of her diet, she found herself adding ketchup to foods she had formerly eaten without it. Frustrated by feeling continually hungry and not losing weight, she finally thought of checking the label on the ketchup bottle. Oops! Four grams per tablespoon—and nobody uses just 1 tablespoon. If you think a tablespoon of ketchup sounds like a lot, I urge you to go and measure it. You will find that it is virtually impossible to use just 1 tablespoon of ketchup; a normal serving, say, the amount you need to cover a burger, is at least 2 tablespoons, and many people, without even realizing it, use 4 or 5 tablespoons.

Just about every condiment has some added sugar or sweetener, so read your labels carefully. (Remember the "Eleven Other Tasty Toxins" on page 64.) When we're thinking about weight loss, we tend to think that condiments don't count—but our belly fat and ravenous hunger say otherwise.

Sugar Saboteurs

- ☐ Ketchup
- ☐ Mustard (except for Dijon mustard)
- ☐ Relish

- ☐ Barbecue sauce
- ☐ Steak sauce
- ☐ Salsa
- ☐ Jams and fruit spreads, including the all-fruit, "all-natural" ones

Appetite-Friendly Alternatives

- ☐ Lemon or lime juice. These are the only two fruit juices you don't have to worry about as long as you use them only as seasonings and *sparingly*—I don't want you making lemonade or limeade, because that will be loaded with simple sugars even if you flavor it with an artificial sweetener. And avoid squeezing lemon slices in your water. It's important to stay well hydrated, but you can inadvertently get a lot of sugar through those lemon squeezes.
- ☐ Olive oil. You will moderate the amount of olive oil you consume later on because of its overall caloric load and the relative ease with which it is consumed, but in Phases 1 and 2 of the Appetite Solution, enjoy up to 3 tablespoons of this delicious healthy fat per meal.
- ☐ Dijon mustard.
- ☐ Avocado. Mashed with some lemon and lime, it adds zest to a piece of grilled chicken or fish or makes a nice side condiment with your steak or burger.
- ☐ Chopped fresh tomatoes, maybe with some coriander, garlic, lemon, and olive oil.
- ☐ Homemade mango salsa (see the recipe on page 260, along with other suggestions for healthy homemade condiments that are quick and easy to prepare).
- ☐ Any type of vinegar—red, white, cider, balsamic, flavored—but check the label to make sure that no sugars have been added.
- ☐ Any fresh or dried herb or spice: garlic, basil, tarragon, oregano, etc.

4. Packaged Cereals

Sugary cereals are an obvious no-no, but even the "nonsweet" cereals are loaded with simple sugars. Special K, for example, has 4 grams in 1 cup of cereal, and Raisin Bran has 20 grams of simple sugars per cup. And that's even before you add the milk! Cream of wheat also has as many as 20 grams of simple sugar per serving. The labels for these products often tend to camouflage the sugars in the carb totals, and some don't even note the number of grams of sugar.

Now, you might go to the store, scrutinize the labels, and find some brands that offer exactly 5 grams of sugar per serving—and you might think you have gotten off scot-free. But think again, because the serving sizes given in nutritional information are often far smaller than the amount most people would typically eat.

For example, Grape-Nuts cereal proclaims that you get only 5 grams of sugars per serving—but a serving is only ½ cup. Measure 4 ounces (115 grams) of cereal into a bowl and tell me whether that looks like enough food to satisfy you for breakfast. I'd still be hungry after eating such a tiny portion, and so would you.

Sugar Saboteurs
☐ Packaged cereals
☐ Granola—usually sweetened with honey or maple syrup
☐ Cream of wheat—and also, watch out for the add-ons, such as milk, raisins, honey, and other sugary sweeteners
☐ Cream of rice—watch out for the add-ons here, too

Appetite-Friendly Alternatives
☐ Homemade unsweetened granola
☐ Porridge—if you eat it plain or dress it with almond milk, fresh fruit, and a sugar substitute rather than cow's milk, raisins, and sugar. You can find almond milk in the dairy section, over to the side of the regular milks.

5. Snack Foods

Like white bread, snack foods such as pretzels, crackers, and crisps are all made from refined flours or starchy foods that might be low in simple sugars but are high in starches. As a result, they are so easily digested that they quickly disrupt your blood sugar and, as a result, your insulin levels. If you are trying to lose weight and transform your appetite from ravenous to pleasant, avoid all snack foods.

Sugar Saboteurs

☐ Pretzels

☐ Crackers

☐ Crisps

Appetite-Friendly Alternatives

☐ Air-popped popcorn

☐ Rice crackers

☐ Toasted wholemeal pita bread

☐ Nuts, such as almonds, walnuts, and cashews

☐ Peanuts—but plain, not honey-roasted. By this point, you can probably detect where the sugar saboteur lurks in a *honey*-roasted peanut!

☐ Raw carrots

☐ Apple slices

☐ Fresh berries

6. Energy Drinks

As many as 27 grams of simple sugars can be found in one 8.4-ounce (250-millilitre) can of Red Bull, to take one popular example. Significantly, the company website tells you that this is comparable to the sugars you would find in an 8.4-ounce (250-millilitre) glass of orange juice—which is why I don't want you drinking orange juice either.

Of course, you can find sugar-free energy drinks, but the caffeine in them can interfere with your sleep, and sleep is crucial for weight loss. (See chapter 4 for more about sleep and the Appetite Solution.)

Sugar Saboteurs

☐ Energy drinks

Appetite-Friendly Alternative
☐ A maximum of 16 ounces (480 millilitres) of your favorite caffeinated beverage, but only before noon to keep it from interfering with your sleep

7. Vitamin Water

Wouldn't you assume that something with the word "vitamin" in its name would be healthy, and something called "water" would be sugar-free?

No on both counts. Vitamin water can have more than 30 grams of simple sugars per 20-ounce (600-millilitre) bottle. It's hard to believe that simple sugars are such a big part of our diet that they show up even in water, but at least now you know how to look for them and protect yourself.

Sugar Saboteur
☐ Vitamin water

Appetite-Friendly Alternative
☐ Plain water

8. Bottled Iced Tea

We don't tend to think of beverages as diet pitfalls, but they often are, even the "healthy" ones: fruit and vegetable juices, vitamin water, and also bottled iced tea—even the "healthy" green tea with honey. You can find un-sweetened or sugar-free bottled ice tea, but most versions of this drink have enough grams of simple sugars to sabotage your weight and inflate your appetite before you've even finished the bottle. To take just one example, there are a full 38 grams of simple sugars in just one bottle of Snapple "all-natural" lemon tea.

Sugar Saboteur
☐ Bottled, sweetened iced tea

Appetite-Friendly Alternative
☐ Unsweetened ice tea, or perhaps iced tea sweetened with your favorite artificial sweetener

9. Packaged and Processed Foods

Even if these don't *seem* sweet, packaged and processed foods almost always contain some form of sweetener to enhance flavor and also to act as a preservative. Of course, these foods frequently include white flour, white potato, and corn as well.

More Sugar Saboteurs Where You'd Never Expect Them

- ☐ Peanut butter: 3 grams of simple sugars per 2 ounces (60 grams), and most people use way more than this
- ☐ Pizza: 3.5 grams of simple sugars per slice—and most people don't stop at one slice
- ☐ Honey-roasted peanuts: 16 grams per ½ cup (70 grams)
- ☐ Fruit rollups: 7 grams per piece
- ☐ Soy milk : 10 grams of simple sugars per cup (240 millilitres), however, unsweetened organic soymilk has only 1 gram per cup
- ☐ Rice milk: 10 grams of simple sugars per cup (240 millilitres)
- ☐ Trail mix: at least 11 grams per ¼ cup (40 grams)—and nobody eats just this amount, which is less than a single handful
- ☐ Flavored cereal bar: 13 to 14 grams per bar
- ☐ Prepared coleslaw: as many as 14 grams of simple sugars
- ☐ Canned baked beans: as many as 18 grams of simple sugars
- ☐ Flavored energy bar: about 21 grams per bar
- ☐ Fast-food chicken sandwich: 21 grams of sugar in one example that included a honey barbecue sauce
- ☐ Protein bars: not all of these are sugar-filled, but many have up to 23 grams or more per bar
- ☐ Dried cranberries: 26 grams per serving (that small ¼-cup serving again)
- ☐ Raisins: 30 grams per ¼-cup (25-gram) serving
- ☐ Flavored coffee drinks: one 16-ounce (480-millilitre) example of a hazelnut macchiato contains 32 grams of simple sugars

The Preparation Spectrum

As we have seen, sometimes a food contains complex carbs when it's raw or lightly cooked, but those complex carbs become simple sugars when the food is baked, boiled, juiced, or blenderized. That's because the cooking or blending does the work that your intestines are supposed to do, liberating the simple sugar from its fiber honeycomb.

Any cooking or preparation that erodes or decays the honeycomb is going to do this before your intestines have the chance. Of course, for your first six weeks of the Appetite Solution, you won't have to worry about planning and preparation much because you will be following my meal plans (see chapter 5), and I've done the thinking for you. However, you might occasionally need to substitute a restaurant meal or even a meal at someone's house for one that I have planned for you, and certainly after the first six weeks, you will be planning your own meals. So here's what you need to know about the Preparation Spectrum:

☐ where along the spectrum a food remains a complex carb that will not challenge your blood sugar, inflate your appetite, or threaten your metabolism, and

☐ at what point it turns into a simple sugar that will trigger an insulin response, set you up for hunger, and cue your body to store fat.

If your primary goal is to reduce simple sugar intake and transform your appetite, "raw" is best. Raw, whole food contains the fewest sugars, and you'll find such food both the most filling and the least likely to trigger sugar cravings.

However, we have other goals related to our food intake: We want to be fully nourished, and we want to enjoy our food. Cooking helps us meet those goals because it doesn't just liberate simple sugars, it also liberates vitamins and nutrients, making them more *bioavailable* (that is, available to our biochemistry). And of course, we love the taste of a baked sweet potato, a stalk of broccoli sautéed lightly with garlic, or a grilled red pepper.

I don't want you to feel even a little bit deprived as you follow the

Appetite Solution; I want you to revel in the delicious tastes and textures of your food. So here's the Preparation Spectrum showing how preparation affects simple sugar content and, therefore, your appetite and metabolism.

Preparations That Create a Healthy, Pleasant Appetite

☐ **Raw** is best.

☐ **Grilled,** because you don't have to use as much oil or engage in the process of frying, which can be mildly inflammatory.

☐ **Sautéed or stir-fried, lightly,** with a small amount of olive oil, which is almost as good as grilling.

☐ **Steamed,** using a steamer basket so that the food never touches boiling water; you want to stop steaming when the vegetables are still firm and almost crunchy, well before they are soggy and limp. Remember, you don't want them to be predigested—you want them firm enough that you have to put some effort into chewing and then digesting them. If it's too easy to eat them, they have lost too much of the fiber that makes them chewy—and complex. By the way, you can steam whole grains also, including rice and quinoa, and you can also steam whole-grain pasta. The same goes for all these foods—don't cook them until they are mushy. They should retain their texture and feel at least a little "tough."

☐ **Baked,** but again, stop before food is mushy. I would recommend against baking fruits, such as apples, which will turn right to sugar when they are soft enough to enjoy. However, if you want to bake a sweet potato or throw some carrots and onions in with a pot roast (once you are planning your own meals), you're still on the safe side. The mushier the food, however, the more simple sugars have been liberated from it, so be aware.

Preparations That Create a Ravenous, Overwhelming Appetite

☐ **Boiling.** Many people cook their vegetables by boiling them, and it's one of the easiest ways to turn a healthy, metabolism-supporting complex carb into a bunch of simple sugars. Also, many of the vitamins and nutrients of vegetables leach out into the water through boiling. You'll notice I don't include any soups during the first six weeks of your meal plan, and I don't recommend that you rely on them or any other type of boiling, which comes far too close to "predigesting" your food and turning otherwise healthy foods into simple sugars.

☐ **Blenderizing.** Feel free to enjoy a protein shake—I include some on my meal plans, and I recommend some in Resources for you to use. But don't throw any fruit into the blender; instead, enjoy fresh, whole fruit on the side. You can also eat frozen fruit, but make sure it was fresh when it was frozen; avoid anything that has been stewed or turned into syrup, jam, or "all-natural" apple butter.

☐ **Juicing.** Juicing a fruit, even a lemon, transforms the complex carbs into simple sugars. You can use lemon or lime juice sparingly as a seasoning, but as I already mentioned: avoid the lemonade. Furthermore, a glass of orange juice is ridiculously full of simple sugars. Why do you think they give it to people whose blood sugar has dropped, such as diabetics in insulin shock or people who have just donated blood? If you *need* a sudden jolt to your blood sugar, orange juice is terrific; but if you're trying to lose weight, transform your appetite, and reset your metabolism, even a single glass of orange juice once a week can really do you in. A lot of diet plans encourage you to consume green juices or to throw some kale into your protein shake, but by now you can see what the problem is with that: The blenderizing predigests these foods and transforms their healthy complex carbs into problematic simple sugars. Stick to the upper end of the Preparation Spectrum and you'll be fine.

The Estrogen Experiment

The "estrogen experiment" is what I call the large-scale plan of many commercial dairy farms to load us up with hormones through their dairy products. Because of the unhealthy or extreme conditions in which most commercial dairy is produced, the cows have to be dosed with antibiotics to combat infection, and they are often pumped full of estrogen to keep them producing milk. Other animals farmed for meat are often loaded with hormones and antibiotics as well.

And guess what? Both hormones and antibiotics are fattening, not to mention other problems that both men and women encounter when they are overloaded with female hormones.

Antibiotics are fattening because they destroy huge swaths of the friendly bacteria that live in our digestive tracts and enable us to digest our food as well as supporting our immune systems and overall health. Farmers know that antibiotics have this weight-stimulating effect because they don't administer them just to animals that are sick—they also do it to fatten them up.

Estrogen has a weight-stimulating effect, too, disrupting your blood sugar levels, metabolism, and appetite. Opt out of this large-scale experiment by avoiding cow's milk, which even before it is dosed with estrogen and antibiotics is already full of simple sugars. Note that skimmed milk contains even more simple sugars because when you take out the fat, sugar is much of what's left.

Ideally, avoid commercially raised beef and chicken as well, focusing on organic, free-range, and grass-fed animals. Organic products can be more expensive, and of course, you won't find simple sugars in your meats, so use your own judgment. But definitely avoid cow's milk, especially since almond milk and coconut milk are such easy and healthy switches.

The Protein Push

One way to combat the effects of simple sugar on your metabolism, your appetite, and your weight is simply to cut back on their consumption—slowly and gradually, so as not to trigger adaptive thermogenesis. At the same time, you can overcome the insidious effects of the sugar saboteurs by loading up your diet with protein, which will both support muscle repair and combat hunger.

The satisfying effect of protein and its beneficial effects on weight loss have been noted in numerous studies. For example, a 2008 article in *Physiology and Behavior,* authored by a team of scientists from Maastricht University in the Netherlands reported that both "satiety" (feelings of fullness) and "energy expenditure" (calorie-burning) were important for weight loss—and that increased protein consumption supported both. The authors concluded that "protein-induced satiety appears to be of vital importance for weight loss and weight maintenance," noting that significantly greater weight loss was observed in experimental subjects given high-protein diets compared with subjects who were not.[24]

A 2014 article suggests some reasons why this might be so.[25] The researchers compared the effects of *ghrelin,* a hormone produced in your stomach that stimulates appetite, with the biochemical effects of a high-protein diet. The biology is intricate, but the takeaway is simple: While ghrelin makes you feel hungry, protein keeps you feeling full. In the battle between ghrelin and protein, protein wins.

A 2014 article by another group of Dutch scientists explored the effects of what they called "protein leverage"—using protein to improve the effectiveness of diets. In a twelve-day study of seventy-nine men and women given diets with 5 percent, 15 percent, and 30 percent protein, the high-protein diets induced subjects to consume fewer calories and to feel less hungry.[26]

Likewise, another 2014 article, which reviewed the latest literature on the topic, found that "a diet rich in high-quality protein is a beneficial dietary strategy to prevent and/or treat obesity."[27]

Enough said! Trust the Appetite Solution and its Phase 1, Push the Protein, to keep you feeling full and satisfied while you make the transition to a lower-calorie diet with a lot fewer simple sugars. You'll be eating lots of protein all through the Appetite Solution, and in chapter 11, I'll show you how to combat the effects of any indulgences using protein as well. Protein is your secret weapon in the battle to transform your appetite and shed excess fat—and lucky for all of us, it's delicious and filling as well!

A Successful Solution

Now that you know *why* the Appetite Solution will work for you, it's time to find out exactly *how* it works. In Part II, you will find a complete explanation of the three phases of the Appetite Solution, your meal plans, and your fitness plans. Get ready to transform your appetite, reset your metabolism on "high," and shed your excess fat. This is the first step in your journey toward achieving a healthy weight and enjoying the metabolism of a teenager.

Part II

Your Six-Week Appetite Solution

Chapter 4

Eat Your Fill for the Next Six Weeks

Now that you know why the Appetite Solution is going to succeed where your other diet plans have failed, it's time to get started on your success! In this chapter, I explain everything that you'll be doing for the next six weeks. In chapter 5, you'll find six weeks' worth of detailed meal plans, along with weekly shopping lists. Any recipes you might need are at the back of this book, starting on page 255. In chapter 6, I'll talk you through my approach to exercise, and then in chapter 7, you'll find detailed fitness plans for Phase 2, Phase 3, and beyond. (As you recall, I don't want you varying your current level of activity while you are still in Phase 1, so as not to trigger adaptive thermogenesis.) I've even developed two different fitness plans: one for those of you who have already been working out, and one for those of you who are just getting started.

In Part III, you'll find additional support for the first six weeks of the Appetite Solution—and beyond. Chapter 8, "Solutions for Every Situation," helps you make the Appetite Solution work when you are eating in restaurants or at someone's home, traveling, or celebrating the holidays. You'll also find a number of supportive tips for eating in this new way. Chapter 9, "Appetite Pitfalls," helps you identify common food-related mistakes that are easy to make—places where my patients and I myself have inadvertently sabotaged our weight-loss efforts without even realizing it. I'm happy to help you learn from *our* mistakes so you don't have to make your own! Chapter 10, "Pushing Past Plateaus," is just what it sounds like: my best advice for what to do if you hit a plateau sometime after your first six weeks of the Appetite Solution. And in chapter 11, "Enjoying the Metabolism of a Teenager," I share with you my special Protein Protocol for indulging in your favorite treats while still keeping your metabolism burning high and hot.

But first things first! Let me talk you through the Appetite Solution so you can begin to reset your metabolism, transform your appetite, and achieve your healthy weight.

The Appetite Solution: An Overview

Note: The calorie totals and percentages do contain some approximations but have been carefully calculated, and any variations are statistically insignificant.

Phase 1, Push the Protein

During Phase 1 of the Appetite Solution, you will consume 2,000 to 2,400 calories per day for two weeks, along with these other points:

Protein: 30–40 percent of daily calories

Fats: 30–40 percent of daily calories

Carbohydrates: 30–40 percent of daily calories

Simple sugars, included in your carbohydrate count: You'll start with 40 grams per day on Day 1 and will bring it down gradually to less than 20 grams per day by Day 14.

Exercise: Continue at your current level, whatever that is.

Eat everything on the meal plans—do not skip meals or omit items!

Phase 2, Shelve the Sugar

During Phase 2 of the Appetite Solution, you will still consume 2,000 to 2,400 calories per day for two weeks, along with a change in your intake of simple sugar and exercise:

Protein: 30–40 percent of daily calories

Fats: 30–40 percent of daily calories

Carbohydrates: 30–40 percent of daily calories

Simple sugars, included in your carbohydrate count: You will consume at most 5 grams per meal or snack for a total of less than 20 grams of simple sugar/day.

Exercise: Begin your Appetite Solution fitness plan for Phase 2. (See chapter 6.)

Eat everything on the meal plans—do not skip meals or omit items!

Phase 3, Shed the Fat

During Phase 3 of the Appetite Solution, you will consume only 2,000 calories per day for two weeks—and beyond—along with these other points:

Protein: 30–40 percent of daily calories

Fats: 30–40 percent of daily calories

Carbohydrates: 30–40 percent of daily calories

Simple sugars, included in your carbohydrate count: You will consume at most 5 grams per meal or snack for a total of less than 20 grams of simple sugar/day.

You may now eat less than is indicated on the meal plans—but never more. If you leave something out of one meal or even skip a meal, eat no more than what is indicated for the next meal or snack.

Treat the Appetite Solution as a Medical Protocol

Throughout the Appetite Solution, I have carefully crafted your balance of protein, fats, and carbohydrates, and I have carefully calibrated your reduction of simple sugars. Because of the way these different food types interact, I want to make sure that you eat enough protein to jam the hunger signal, enough complex carbs to support your energy, and enough healthy fats to nourish your brain and balance your mood. Although your own natural hunger will eventually direct you to the foods that you know your body needs, you will not yet be at that point when you begin Phase 1.

So I'm going to request that you follow my protocol to the letter during Phases 1 and 2. If I ask you to eat 8 ounces (230 grams) of fish at a meal, please eat all of it—don't stop partway through. If I suggest that you eat two slices of wholemeal toast, don't decide that you'd rather "go low-carb" and skip the bread.

I also want you to start with the protein at every meal. If you are simply unable to eat everything I recommend, it is most important that you eat all the protein. If you don't, your appetite and your metabolism will remain off balance, and this weight-loss program might not work for you.

If you're reading this book, it's because your appetite and metabolism haven't worked so far. You need a boost, and I'm delighted to give you one—but if my approach is going to give you the success you deserve, you need to follow my recommendations to the letter and eat everything I suggest. Please consider this eating plan a medical protocol, and follow it as you would a prescription.

"Plug and Play"

I *do* want you to follow the Appetite Solution to the letter—but I *don't* want you to feel restricted. So here's what I've done.

During Phases 2 and 3, just about every meal and snack can be swapped out for another meal or snack of the same type from the same phase. In other words, switch out any Phase 2 breakfast with any other Phase 2 breakfast. Switch out any Phase 2 midmorning snack with any other Phase 2 midmorning snack. And so on. Don't switch a breakfast with a lunch, and don't switch a Phase 2 meal with a Phase 3 meal. But if you stick within meal type and phase, you can switch as you like.

There are five breakfasts where I went a little wild and gave you some extra treats. Those are the *only* meals I don't want you swapping, or you might end up getting too many calories by the end of the week. I've labeled those "Treat Meals," so you'll remember not to swap them. Any other meals, however, you can swap within the phase.

But please *don't* switch individual items. I've worked hard to balance every nutritional need at each meal and to make sure each meal affects your metabolism and your appetite in a positive way. If I suggest blueberries in one meal and an apple in another, please don't switch the blueberries with the apple. It sounds like a trivial switch, but while you are trying to reset your appetite and your metabolism, these kinds of changes can really throw the whole plan off, keeping you from achieving the success that you deserve.

And of course, please follow Phase 1 exactly as I present it. During Phase 1, I'm slowly cutting back on your simple sugars in a way that will foil adaptive thermogenesis and avoid a stress response. If you start making changes during Phase 1, you could sabotage your success for the whole program.

Buy Kitchen Scales

When you follow the Appetite Solution, you are getting used to a whole new way of eating. Eventually, you'll be able to cook and eat "by feel," but when you first get started, you won't necessarily have a sense of the portion sizes I recommend.

For you to ensure maximum success, I'd like you to invest in kitchen scales—you can find one for $25 (about £15) or less—as well as a set of measuring cups and spoons. I'd also like you to commit to measuring *everything,* especially condiments. Remember, a regular small spoon is not the same size as a "teaspoon," and a large soup spoon usually holds far more than a "tablespoon." Nor is a coffee cup or glass equivalent to an 8-ounce (240-millilitre) cup. So please use actual measuring cups and spoons to measure.

Please don't assume you know how much "2 tablespoons" of ketchup is until you've measured it out several times for several weeks. You will be tempted to sneak in a little more—maybe even a lot more—of the high-sugar foods, especially as you are starting to cut back on simple sugars. I suggest that you carry an extra set of measuring spoons in your handbag or pocket, so you can be sure not to overdo the creamer in your coffee or the oil on your salad.

You will also be tempted to eat less of the proteins and complex carbs that you might not be used to, and then your metabolism, your appetite, and your weight will not respond properly.

Once you've finished six weeks of the Appetite Solution, you'll be super-comfortable with the measurements we're using. At that point, if you want to prepare meals by feel, be my guest. However, if you notice that you've started regaining a few pounds, you might want to go back and check your measurements again. When I tell you that even I have gained some extra weight by making some mistakes in this department, you'll see how easy, and how dangerous, it can be to mis-measure. (To read that story, check out chapter 9.)

Summary of the Appetite Solution Protocol

Phase 1: Eat everything on the plan, starting with the protein. If you physically can't eat all the food I recommend, make sure you at least consume the protein.

Phase 2: Eat everything on the plan, starting with the protein. Feel free to swap any meal on this phase with another meal of the same type—that is, any Phase 2 breakfast for any other Phase 2 breakfast, any Phase 2 midmorning snack with any other Phase 2 midmorning snack, etc. But do not swap individual items—for instance, one type of fruit for another.

Phase 3: Follow your natural hunger if you want to eat *less*, but never eat *more* than is recommended by the plan. Swap any Phase 3 meal with any other Phase 3 meal of the same type—for instance, any Phase 3 breakfast with any other Phase 3 breakfast. Do not swap individual items.

Buy kitchen scales and a set of measuring cups and spoons, and measure *everything*.

Goals for Phase 1

The beginning of an eating plan is often the hardest. Any type of change can be challenging, and changes in what you eat—such a personal and emotional issue for most people—are often the most challenging of all. I want to make the Appetite Solution as easy as possible for you, both to ensure your success and because anything stressful is likely to trigger a stress response, which will only make it harder for you to lose weight.

Phase 1 is when we start to transform your appetite from overwhelming and uncomfortable to easy and pleasant. So here are my goals for you during Phase 1:

- ☐ *Keep you from triggering either adaptive thermogenesis or a stress response.* I don't want your body to think it's starving, and I don't want to stress you out. Both of these outcomes will only cue your body to conserve energy and store fat, and both will inflate your appetite as your body tries to get you to eat extra calories to make up for the ones you've cut back on. So during Phase 1, you're consuming a higher number of calories than you will consume later on. You're also eating quite a bit of protein to foil adaptive thermogenesis and to jam the hunger signals. High protein consumption will keep your body out of "starvation mode," and it will keep you from feeling hungry by the time you reach Day 4, or maybe even sooner.
- ☐ *Start decreasing your consumption of simple sugars.* Remember, your blood sugar levels are raised by consuming both too many simple sugars in one meal and too many simple sugars in the course of a day. The Magic Rule of 5 and 20 says that you can have up to 5 grams of simple sugars per meal or snack, for a total of up to 20 grams of simple sugars per day. By the time you reach the end of Phase 1, you will have reached that goal.
- ☐ *Transform your appetite.* Many factors during Phase 1 will help to dissolve your hunger: your relatively high intake of calories, your consumption of complex carbs and healthy fats, and, most importantly, your high consumption of protein. By Day 4, you won't feel hungry at all, and many of you will stop feeling hungry well before that.

During Phase 1, I make sure you are consuming plenty of calories, with lots of complex carbohydrates and healthy fats to keep you feeling full. Most important, you will be consuming a high percentage of your daily calories in protein, which jams the hunger signal in your brain, foils adaptive thermogenesis, and short-circuits the stress response. Protein also protects your muscle, allowing your body to repair any damage or strain.

Meanwhile, you've also cut back on simple sugars, which will set you up for weight loss during Phases 2 and 3. My goal is for you to lose fifteen pounds (close to 7 kilos) or half your excess weight by the end of Phase 3—to lose that weight, and to keep it off, easily, for life. My ultimate goal is for you to lose all your excess weight and to achieve the metabolism of a teenager so that you can indulge in a few more treats once in a while without risking your healthy weight. And throughout this whole process, my goal is for you to feel full and satisfied, experiencing only mild, pleasant hunger and not the devastating or overwhelming kind.

I know you can achieve these goals, because I've seen thousands of my patients do so. I'm honestly not too worried about whether you lose weight during Phase 1, though some of you will lose a little. But if we *start* by looking for quick weight loss, guess what will happen? Because it takes between five and fourteen days to reset your metabolism and get it to start burning fat, any dramatic weight loss before then is almost certainly going to be muscle plus water, and it is almost certainly going to be temporary.

I've seen it time and time again: Going for the quick weight loss invariably does more harm than good, so during Phase 1, that is not our focus. You will enjoy a burst of energy during Phase 1, a better mood, a clearer brain, better memory, and very likely (as many of my patients have told me) a better sex life. Your skin will be clearer, your hair will thicken and be healthier, you'll sleep better, and you'll notice how much better you look, regardless of what the scale says. And of course, you won't be hungry.

Goals for Phase 2

By the time you start Phase 2, you're down to a healthy level of simple sugars—a level that is going to enable you to reset your metabolism, transform your appetite, and lose weight. During Phase 2, although your calorie consumption is still a bit high, your simple sugar consumption now follows the Magic Rule of 5 and 20: no more than 5 grams of simple sugar per meal or snack, and a total of no more than 20 grams of simple sugar per day.

As in Phase 1, you'll be consuming lots of complex carbs and healthy fats, which will keep you feeling full, as well as lots of protein, which will continue to jam the hunger signals. During Phase 2 you will also begin your

Appetite Solution fitness plan—either my Chelsea Plan, for those of you who are new to exercise, or my Martina Plan, for those of you who are more experienced (see chapter 7, "Your Appetite Solution Fitness Plan").

Adding exercise makes protein consumption even more important. Your body uses protein to build muscle—and building muscle gives you an incredible metabolic boost.

As in Phase 1, please be sure to eat everything on your Phase 2 meal plans. For the Appetite Solution to reset your metabolism and transform your appetite, you need to follow it to the letter. Cutting out portions of the meal plans could potentially sabotage all your efforts.

So here are my goals for you during Phase 2:

☐ *Continue to foil adaptive thermogenesis and the stress response.* We add in exercise only after your body has gotten used to its new way of eating—and we add it slowly and gradually.

☐ *Stay at a low consumption of simple sugars to facilitate weight loss.* We got you here gradually, but now you *are* here, at a healthy low level of simple sugars that will allow your blood insulin levels to decline as well. Lower blood insulin levels cue your body to burn fat instead of storing it—and the weight loss begins!

☐ *Begin building lean muscles.* Lean muscles are the best gift you can give to your metabolism. Remember, the higher proportion of lean muscle you have, the higher and hotter your metabolism burns. People with a high proportion of lean muscle burn more calories even when they are sleeping compared with people who have a higher proportion of body fat. Exercise will help you develop the lean muscles that eventually help you achieve the metabolism of a teenager.

☐ *Maintain a pleasant appetite.* Your relatively high intake of calories and your high consumption of protein—along with your consumption of complex carbs and healthy fats—will keep you from feeling hungry.

Goals for Phase 3

Here is one of the big milestones for Phase 3: Your appetite will now be responding to all the healthy changes you have been making, and you will start to notice that you are often less hungry than you are used to being. So at this point, if you want to eat *less* than the meal plan calls for, you can—as long as you don't eat *more* at the next meal. Allow your natural hunger to take over, but don't fall into the trap of skipping meals and then overeating. Eating *less* at a meal but never *more* will help you discover your healthy appetite.

By the time you reach Phase 3, you will be losing three to five pounds (about 1.5 to 2 kilos) per week. Your appetite will be mild and pleasant, your metabolism will be humming, and you will enjoy clearer thinking, a better mood, and way more energy than you have probably experienced for a long time. So here are my goals for you during Phase 3:

☐ *Continue to foil adaptive thermogenesis and the stress response.* Now that your body is used to exercise and this approach to eating, we can cut calories down to an optimal 2,000 per day.

☐ *Stay at a low consumption of simple sugars to facilitate weight loss.* As long as you need to lose excess fat, you should be able to drop three to five pounds (about 1.5 to 2 kilos) per week because of your low consumption of simple sugars.

☐ *Continue building lean muscles.* The higher your proportion of muscle to fat, the closer you are to achieving the metabolism of a teenager.

☐ *Maintain a pleasant appetite.* Now that your body is used to this way of eating, your metabolism is humming, and your hunger is just what it needs to be in order to maintain your healthy weight.

Phase 3 is the final phase of the six-week eating plan, and it's also your lifetime maintenance plan. For as long as you still need to lose weight, following the principles of Phase 3 will help you accomplish that goal. Once you have achieved your healthy weight, remaining on Phase 3 will keep you there. In chapter 11, I explain how you can occasionally indulge during Phase 3, once you have achieved the weight loss you were seeking.

Simple Sugars Where You'd Least Expect Them: Condiments, Sauces, and Creamers

As you saw in chapter 3, simple sugars lurk in all sorts of unexpected places, including tomato sauce and such condiments as ketchup and barbecue sauce. I know that many people love these foods and condiments, and I want you to enjoy yourself when you are following the Appetite Solution while also cutting back on your simple sugars and achieving a healthy weight. So here's the deal I'd like to make with you:

☐ You promise to measure every single sauce and condiment, using only the amounts I specify on this plan.

☐ I'll include *some* sauces and condiments, in amounts low enough to hold to the Magic Rule of 5 and 20, with no more than 5 grams of simple sugar per meal or snack, and no more than 20 grams of simple sugar by the end of the day.

I want you to keep an eagle eye out for all those little extra places where simple sugars lurk and never to think that a food "doesn't count." Here are three common pitfalls—foods that people consume without realizing that they add to the simple sugar count:

☐ *Skimmed milk.* Just because something is merely added to your coffee doesn't mean that it doesn't count as a food—and as we have seen, skimmed milk is super-high in simple sugars. Soy and rice milk are also high in simple sugars, so please avoid them, too. Substitute either unsweetened almond milk or unsweetened coconut milk, and don't use more than 2 ounces (60 millilitres) per cup of coffee. There are 2 tablespoons (6 teaspoons) in every ounce (30 millilitres), so please, carry a measuring spoon with you and measure carefully. (See "What Are You Drinking?," pages 93–94 for more.)

☐ *Coffee creamers.* Creamers come in many varieties, and some of them are quite high in sugar, especially the flavored, fat-free dairy creamers. If you use a coffee creamer instead of almond or coconut milk, make sure you use one that is sugar free and doesn't contain any high-fructose corn syrup or other caloric sweeteners. And again, no more than 2 ounces (4 tablespoons) per cup of coffee.

☐ *Salad dressings.* Salad dressings can be quite high in sugar, especially the fat-free variety. Please avoid them. When you prepare your meals at home, make your own dressings (I include directions in this book). If you eat at a restaurant or in someone else's home, ask for olive oil and either vinegar or some lemon and dress your own salad. You don't want salad to be the place where your weight loss gets sabotaged—but if you rely on prepared dressings, that's exactly the risk you run.

Simple Sugars Versus Complex Carbohydrates

As you saw in Part I, the same food can be either a complex carb or a simple sugar, depending on how it is prepared.

Complex Carbs	Simple Sugars
Fresh, whole fruit	Juiced, stewed, baked, blenderized, packaged, canned, dried, zip-locked, or vacuum-packed fruit
Fresh frozen fruit (but check for additives)	Fruit included in flavored yogurt
Raw, grilled, or lightly sautéed tomatoes	Juiced or stewed tomatoes; tomato sauce
Raw, grilled, or lightly sautéed vegetables	Juiced or stewed vegetables

For all three phases of the Appetite Solution, you don't have to worry about counting simple sugars because I've done that for you. However, if you are eating at a restaurant or at someone's house or you're traveling (see chapter 8), you might need to figure out whether a meal has too many simple sugars.

If you're in that situation, here's your shortcut: Don't worry about the sugars in fruits and vegetables that are fresh, grilled, or lightly sautéed. But avoid completely any form of fruit or vegetable that is juiced, stewed, baked, or blenderized, even if there is just a little bit of it, as in a sauce or salad dressing.

If you're buying prepared or packaged foods, look at both the nutrition information (where they show the number of calories, carbs, sugars, etc.) and the ingredients. Don't worry about the sugar content if you see that all the ingredients are fresh, grilled, or lightly sautéed vegetables or fruits. Quite possibly, the nutrition information on the label will list lots of sugars—but they'll be the type of sugar you don't have to worry about.

However, if the prepared or packaged food contains any of the following ingredients, avoid it if the label shows more than 5 grams of sugar:

- ☐ Any of the sweeteners listed on page 65
- ☐ Corn
- ☐ White flour or white rice

Weight Loss Through Supplements: Multivitamins and Vitamin D

You should be getting most of your nutrients from food, but I do want you to take a multivitamin and 1,000 milligrams of vitamin D per day. (See Resources for some suggested brands.) Vitamins are a potent source of anti-inflammatory chemicals and antioxidants—biochemicals that combat the oxidative (oxygen-related) stress caused by normal wear and tear. As an extra bonus, they also seem to play a role in helping to prevent cancer.

As we have seen, inflammation is a major contributor to both weight gain and an inflated appetite. For the most part, I'm bringing down your inflammation and combating stress by having you cut back on simple sugars and cutting out alcohol (see below). The vitamins will add nicely to that momentum.

What Are You Drinking?

While you are following the Appetite Solution, I want you to stay well-hydrated—and I don't want you to end up drinking all your calories. So here's your protocol:

☐ Drink at least 64 ounces (about 2 litres) of liquids a day.

☐ Of those, up to 16 ounces (480 millilitres) can be a caffeinated beverage—coffee, tea, or sugar-free caffeinated soda—but please end your caffeine consumption by noon. I want to protect your sleep, which is crucial for weight loss. No energy drinks, please—they are so much more powerful than other caffeinated choices that they might disrupt your sleep even when you drink them in the morning.

☐ Here's a list of acceptable beverages:

- Water
- No-calorie flavored water
- Herb tea
- Decaffeinated tea or coffee—but sweetened only with a zero-calorie sweetener, and add only unsweetened almond or coconut milk, no more than 2 ounces (4 tablespoons) per cup.
- Any zero-calorie diet beverage

☐ Here's a list of beverages to avoid:

- Cow's milk
- Energy drinks
- Fizzy drinks or other drinks that contain calories, including vitamin water, bottled iced tea, and coffee drinks of all types
- Alcohol in any form

Please don't flavor your water with lemon or lime. Remember, fruit juices contain lots of simple sugars—and that includes lemon and lime juice. If you like flavored water, buy the zero-calorie kind.

Alcohol: Don't Drink Your Calories!

The following drinks are considered equivalent in terms of alcohol, but they can vary in the amount of calories they contain:

1½ ounces (45 millilitres) of distilled liquor: 100 calories

5 ounces (150 millilitres) of wine: 100–130 calories

One 12-ounce (350-millilitre) light beer: 100 calories

One 12-ounce (350-millilitre) regular beer: 200 calories

Alcohol: Your Weight-Loss Enemy

If you want to lose weight and control your appetite, alcohol is off the menu. I know that a lot of myths out there say you can make one or two glasses of wine per day part of a healthy diet, but I've got to tell you: It's just not true.

Perhaps you've read about a magical substance called *resveratrol*, a chemical found in the skin of red grapes that when given to mice helped to reduce the risk of obesity, inflammation, diabetes, heart disease, and certain types of cancer. Unfortunately, to realize any of the potential benefits from resveratrol, you would have to drink far more red wine than could ever be considered safe. Fortunately, it can now be found in supplement form without the cork.

There is also a body of scientific literature suggesting that moderate consumption of alcohol (which is not always clearly defined) can benefit your heart. If true, this effect may be related to an alteration in cholesterol metabolism via a net increase in the "good" cholesterol (HDL) and a decrease in the "bad" cholesterol (LDL). Some studies have also suggested that moderate alcohol consumption can lead to a lower incidence of vascular plaque buildup and blood clot formation. Whatever the validity of these studies, they have not persuaded physicians to prescribe any form of alcohol consumption to prevent or treat heart disease or any other medical condition.

In fact, alcohol is a hazardous drug for a number of reasons. It can alter the metabolism of other medications that you might be taking and is especially dangerous when mixed with blood thinners, including aspirin. Chronic or even moderate alcohol use carries substantially more risk to your overall health—high blood pressure, elevated triglyceride levels, numerous cancers, damage to your heart muscle, liver damage resulting in cirrhosis, and the risk of addiction—than any potential benefit.[28]

Many of these problems are even worse if you are overweight or obese. Alcohol can promote frequent and resistant weight gain. Consuming alcohol stimulates your appetite, contributes to dehydration, and increases the amount of calories you eat.

Moreover, even though it is apparently low in sugar, alcohol behaves like a sugar drink. For example, although beer contains no simple sugar, it is loaded with carbohydrates that behave like sugar once you imbibe. And the carbs and sugar in any type of alcoholic beverage get preferential treatment from the liver before it metabolizes any other carbs and fats that are already in your bloodstream. This produces an exaggerated insulin response, with another spin of the sugar cycle, a dip in your blood sugar, and an increase in appetite.

Alcohol also relaxes your central nervous system, which often means that you're paying way less attention to what you eat. If you spend the night drinking and end up having breakfast at 2:00 A.M., the sugar-imbalancing effects of alcohol cause you to crave sugary foods that are likely to inflate your appetite.

Meanwhile, because alcohol behaves like a diuretic—a substance that makes your kidneys generate more urine than is appropriate—you're likely to become dehydrated. Dehydration creates a stress response, which, as we have seen, cues your body to store fat.

Alcohol is directly toxic to your lean muscle tissue and serves to further impair muscle repair and regrowth. It also interferes with the way that other hormones, such as testosterone and naturally occurring human growth hormone, help your body repair and build muscle. Since we want to boost your metabolism by building up lean muscle mass, alcohol is clearly a major obstacle to that process.

Alcohol is also toxic to your liver, which further disrupts your metabolism. Through a chain of biological processes, alcohol raises the level of estrogen in your bloodstream, and the enzymes that would have helped you metabolize carbs and fats are preoccupied with metabolizing the estrogen instead. As a result, your blood lipids increase, and you convert more carbs to body fat. This increased estrogen also puts you at greater risk for a number of types of cancer.

In fact, a study by the National Cancer Institute revealed that in 2009, about 3.5 percent of all cancer deaths in the United States were alcohol-related. For men, alcohol increases the risk of oral, pharyngeal, and laryngeal cancer, as well as cancer of the esophagus. For women, alcohol raises the risk of estrogen-related breast cancers, with alcohol being responsible for 15 percent of all breast cancer deaths occurring in 2009. You don't need to drink much to be at risk: 33 percent of the deaths in the alcohol-related group occurred in people who consumed on average only one drink per day.[29]

As you can see, alcohol's effects on your weight and appetite don't relate only to the liquor itself but also to the way it is consumed and to the other body changes it produces—effects that are rarely included in studies of alcohol and weight.

Having said all that, the research does suggest that when lean individuals consume less than two drinks per day, their weight is not much affected, although there is a slight trend toward being heavier. However, when either overweight or lean people consume more than two drinks per day, significant weight problems result.[30]

Whether by promoting your appetite, relaxing your ability to refrain from that one extra bite, making you thirsty, or boosting your estrogen, alcohol is a weight-management catastrophe that ultimately does nothing for your health. If you are battling your waistline and drinking alcohol, you are further stacking the odds against yourself. For the six weeks of the Appetite Solution, avoid alcohol completely.

Sleep Your Way Thin

Our world is sleep-deprived. Some studies suggest that, here in America, up to 70 million of us don't get enough sleep.[31] This trend is closely associated with the escalation of the worldwide obesity epidemic. Have you ever noticed how much hungrier you are when you are tired? And have you noticed that you're most hungry for starches and simple sugars? It's the sugar cycle on warp drive!

Why does this happen? Well, as we've seen, under stress, your body makes cortisol, which imbalances your blood sugar and also promotes fat storage. And lack of sleep is most definitely a major stressor. If you could do only one thing to help you lose excess fat, getting adequate sleep—from 7½ to 9 hours each night—would probably be your best choice.

Another important thing that happens while you sleep is that your body switches from carbohydrate metabolism to fat metabolism—that is, it stops burning carbs and starts burning fat for energy. This makes sense, because while you're asleep, you can't eat, so your blood sugar drops and your body makes up for it by burning fat. If your body could make you hungry enough to wake you up and send you out foraging for more carbs, it probably would, but most healthy bodies don't operate that way. So during your sleeping hours, you are actually burning fat—and if you don't sleep enough, you burn *less* fat.

I'll give it to you straight: Without 7½ to 9 hours of sleep each night, nothing in your body is functioning normally. If you want the Appetite Solution to work for you, getting enough sleep is mandatory.

How to Improve Your Sleep

☐ Use the bedroom *only* for sleeping and sex: no television, no reading, and particularly, no computer or smartphone; the light of the screens stimulates the part of your brain that keeps you awake.

☐ Avoid bright light sources for at least half an hour before you want to fall asleep, including all electronic screens (TV, computer, phone) and fluorescent lights.

☐ Alcohol is a major sleep disruptor, so here is another reason to avoid it. While a drink might initially make you sleepy, once your liver burns off the alcohol, you often wake up, perhaps in the middle of the night, and your natural sleep cycles are broken. Alcohol also inhibits the refreshing deep sleep (REM sleep, or rapid eye movement) that you really need.

The Sleep Apnea Connection

Let me ask you three simple questions:

☐ Are you waking up more tired than when you went to bed?
☐ Are you often tired during the day—craving a nap or dozing off, even though you've had a full night's sleep?
☐ Do you snore? (Most people don't know if they do, so ask someone who has been with you while you sleep!)

If you answer yes to any of these questions, you might have *sleep apnea,* one of the most underdiagnosed medical conditions in our society.

It is often associated with being overweight, and I see it every day in my practice.

Sleep apnea is characterized by multiple brief waking episodes during sleep. As the muscles around your airway relax, excess tissue surrounding that airway prevents it from opening. Your blood oxygen level drops, and you wake up in order to breathe. Then you go right back to sleep again, unaware that you were ever awake. When you get up in the morning, however, you are sleep-deprived, even if you spent the right amount of time in bed. And, as we just saw, your lack of sleep is unbalancing your blood sugar, inflating your appetite, and cuing your body to store fat.

If you think you might have sleep apnea, talk to your physician. The good news is that as you return to a healthy weight, your sleep apnea might spontaneously clear up on its own.

Stressful Disruptors

As you've seen, feeling stressed is a biological condition that, among other things, inflates your appetite, disrupts your metabolism, and cues your body to store fat.

But stress is also a part of life, and many of the things that stress us are beyond our control. If you're struggling with a difficult situation at work, challenges in a relationship, problems with a child or family member, or any other stressor, that is a part of your life—and yet, you still want to lose weight! So what can you do?

A fabulous stress-reliever while you are following the Appetite Solution is to get the support of a "weight-loss buddy." Check in with each other and keep each other on track. Help each other over the bumps and cheer for each other's successes. You might even enlist the support of a flatmate or spouse, perhaps to exercise with you when you get to Phases 2 and 3.

Meanwhile, if you are stressed, challenged, or overwhelmed, be as compassionate to yourself as you can be. Many of my patients beat themselves up for being stressed—which just stresses them out more! And if they agonize that all the extra stress is making it harder for them to lose weight, then that's *more* stress. Accepting what you cannot change is easier said than done, but see whether you can be loving and compassionate to yourself instead of beating yourself up.

I also suggest that you discover what kinds of support are available. Maybe you can draw on friends, family, or any communities, religious groups, or organizations that you are a part of. If you are the main person responsible for child care in your family, maybe you and a neighbor can trade off some child-care responsibilities so that you both get some kid-free hours each week. Maybe a loved one would be delighted to help with a specific challenge or just be available for a supportive phone call. Often, when we're stressed, we turn inward—but sometimes, looking outward is best.

Finally, try to give yourself at least fifteen stress-free minutes each day, in whatever way works for you. Many of my patients find meditation helpful. Some do yoga. Here are some other "me-time" stress relievers that might work for you:

- ☐ Take a short walk.
- ☐ Sit quietly and listen to some music that you love.
- ☐ "Dance it out"—put on your favorite song and dance like no one is watching!
- ☐ Read a delicious book.
- ☐ Take a warm bath or shower.
- ☐ Watch a TV show you love—but really focus on it, and allow yourself to fully be absorbed by it.
- ☐ Make a "to do" list.
- ☐ Step away from your desk and drink some water.

If you feel that the stress level in your life is more than you are happy about, consider seeking the help of a counselor, therapist, or religious leader. Sometimes what we really need is the perspective that comes from talking to someone who is not part of our daily lives. An outsider can sometimes see solutions that we have missed or offer a perspective that we couldn't get to on our own. Sometimes, too, it's great to vent to a sympathetic ear, someone who won't judge us or expect anything from us.

I wish I could be available to every one of you who is reading this book, so I could talk to you when you're having a bad moment, as I do with my patients. Since that isn't possible, I offer you support through my website (www.drjoecolella.com), where you can find my latest weight-loss suggestions, keep up with the latest research, and even post questions.

In addition, I'd love for you to find another supportive person who will be there for you to help you through the challenges and join you in celebrating your ultimate success!

Set Yourself Up for Success

☐ Drink at least 64 ounces (about 2 litres) of sugar-free liquids every day.

☐ Stick to at most 16 ounces (480 millilitres) of caffeinated liquids, consumed before noon.

☐ Avoid alcohol completely.

☐ Get 7½ to 9 hours of sleep each night.

☐ Get the emotional support you need.

☐ Find ways to de-stress.

Getting Started

And now you're ready to begin! I'm excited for you and the success that I know you can achieve. You're going to feel full and satisfied very soon, and you will love seeing the excess fat come off as your body becomes leaner and your appetite is transformed. Down the road, the ultimate prize is just waiting for you—the metabolism of a teenager. You can absolutely get there, step by step—so let's get started!

Chapter 5

Your Appetite Solution Meal Plans

The following forty-two detailed daily meal plans—six weeks, seven days a week—are the keys to your success. Follow them as discussed in chapter 4. I also include weekly shopping lists to simplify your introduction to the Appetite Solution and help guarantee your success.

Remember that during the three phases of the Appetite Solution, protein, fats, and carbohydrates should count as 30 to 40 percent of your daily calories (with sugars included in the carbohydrate count). At the end of each table you'll see calorie counts and percentages for each of these three categories so you can see how you're sticking to the Appetite Solution guidelines.

Please note that all drinks other than protein shakes should be sugar free—water or artificially sweetened.

> **NOTE**
> In these tables, C. is a cup (240 millilitres), T. is a tablespoon (15 millilitres) and t. is a teaspoon (5 millilitres).

Phase 1/Week 1 Shopping List

Zero-sugar protein powder (such as Isopure brand)

Six medium bananas

1 gallon (4 litres) skimmed milk (lactose-free with calcium)

One jar natural peanut butter

Eight medium apples

1 pound (450 grams) almonds

One jar low-fat mayonnaise

Two medium avocados

Four cans white tuna in water

Four medium tomatoes

One box low-sugar whole-wheat crackers

1 pound (450 grams) whole-wheat pasta

Fresh green beans

1 pound (450 grams) low-fat butter

Six 20–23-gram protein bars (such as Pure Protein brand)

One box reduced-sugar instant porridge

One large orange

One medium orange

Fresh strawberries

Ingredients for turkey chili (recipe page 256)

Parmesan cheese (grated, or you can grate it yourself)

Fresh grapes

Four 8-ounce (230-gram) salmon fillets

12-ounces (340-grams) low-fat (1%) cottage cheese

Three medium peaches

One fresh watermelon

Twelve medium eggs

One loaf wholemeal bread

Two 6-ounce (170-gram) and two 8-ounce (230-gram) skinless chicken breasts

One can small black olives

1½ pounds (700 grams) fresh scallops

16-ounce (450-gram) jar tomato pasta sauce (low-sugar if possible), or see Joe's Tgio sauce (recipe page 258)

Fresh peppers—orange and red are preferred

Two medium lemons

16 ounces (450 grams) smoked salmon

One 2-ounce (60-gram) fillet steak

Two 8-ounce (230-gram) fillet steaks

Wholemeal bagels or wholemeal English muffins

One small jar sliced dill pickles

Two 5-ounce (150-gram) veal chops

One bottle low-sugar barbecue sauce

One bottle sugar-free caramel syrup

One can sundried tomato pesto sauce (low-sugar)

One can sundried tomatoes

Six slices deli roast beef or turkey

One bag coleslaw

Phase 1/Week 1 Daily Menus

DAY 1

	Calories	Fat (g)	Carbs (g)	Protein (g)	Sugar (g)	Simple Sugar (g)
Breakfast						
25-g protein shake	100	0	0	25	0	0
½ banana	52.5	0	13.5	0.5	7	7
1 C. (240 ml) skimmed milk (always okay to swap almond milk with skimmed milk anywhere in the plan)	86	0	12	8	12	12
1 T. peanut butter	100	8	3	4	1.5	1.5

	Calories	Fat (g)	Carbs (g)	Protein (g)	Sugar (g)	Simple Sugar (g)
½ C. (70 g) ice (12 oz./350 ml liquid total in shake)						
8-oz. (240 ml) caffeinated or decaf coffee or tea, or water	0	0	0	0	0	
Breakfast totals	**338.5**	**8**	**28.5**	**37.5**	**20.5**	**20.5**
Midmorning Snack						
1 medium apple, sliced	72	0	19	0	14	
¼ C. (30 g) almonds	206	18	7	8	2	
8-oz. (240 ml) decaf drink						
Snack totals	**278**	**18**	**26**	**8**	**16**	**0**
Lunch						
1 C. (200 g) tuna salad made with 1 T. low-fat mayo	383	10	14.5	30	2	2
½ avocado	160	15	9	2	0	
1 medium tomato, sliced	22	0	5	1	3	
4 whole-wheat crackers	72	3	10	1.5	0	
16-oz. (480 ml) decaf drink						
Lunch totals	**637**	**28**	**38.5**	**34.5**	**5**	**2**
Dinner						
1 C. (115 g) whole-wheat, spaghetti, cooked	124	1	37	7.5	1	
(with 1 T. extra-virgin olive oil)	119	14	0	0	0	
Two 2-inch (5-cm) beef meatballs	228	9	8	27.5	0	
1 C. (240 ml) tomato pasta sauce	185	6	28	5	22	22
1 C. (90 g) fresh green beans	34	0	8	2	1.5	
1 slice wholemeal bread	128	2	24	4	2	
(with 1 t. butter)	33	3.5	0	0	0	
½ C. (60 g) blueberries	41.5	0	11	0.5	7	
16-oz. (480-ml) decaf drink						
Dinner totals	**892.5**	**35.5**	**116**	**46.5**	**33.5**	**22**
Evening Snack						
20-g protein bar (<3g sugar)	200	6	16	20	2	2
8-oz. (240-ml) decaf drink	0	0	0	0	0	
Snack totals	**200**	**6**	**16**	**20**	**2**	**2**

	Calories	Fat (g)	Carbs (g)	Protein (g)	Sugar (g)	Simple Sugar (g)
Day 1 totals	2,342 cal	85.5 g	225 g	146.5 g	77 g	46.5 g
		770 cal	900 cal	586 cal		
Percentage of daily calories		33%	38%	25%		

DAY 2

	Calories	Fat (g)	Carbs (g)	Protein (g)	Sugar (g)	Simple Sugar (g)
Breakfast						
1 C. (240 ml) reduced-sugar instant porridge, cooked	145	2	25	6	2	2
1 sliced medium banana	105	0	27	1	14	
½ C. (120 ml) skimmed milk (always okay to swap almond milk with skimmed milk anywhere in the plan)	43	0	6	4	6	6
1 medium orange	62	0	15	1	12	
12-oz. (350-ml) caffeinated or decaf coffee or tea, or water						
Breakfast totals	**355**	**2**	**73**	**12**	**34**	**8**
Midmorning Snack						
50-g protein shake	200	0	0	50	0	
½ C. (120 ml) skimmed milk (always okay to swap almond milk with skimmed milk anywhere in the plan)	43	0	6	4	6	6
½ C. (60 g) strawberries	26	0	7	0.5	4	
¼ C. (35 g) ice						
12-oz. (350-ml) decaf drink						
Snack totals	**269**	**0**	**13**	**54.5**	**10**	**6**
Lunch						
1 C. (225 g) beef or turkey chili	256	8	22	25	5	5
made with ⅛ C. (20 g) spinach	7	0	1	1	0	
1 T. Parmesan cheese	22	1.4	0	2	0	
4 whole-wheat crackers	76	3	11	1.5	0	
1 C. (100 g) grapes	110	0.3	29	1	25	
16-oz. (480-ml) decaf drink						
Lunch totals	**471**	**12.7**	**63**	**30.5**	**30**	**5**

	Calories	Fat (g)	Carbs (g)	Protein (g)	Sugar (g)	Simple Sugar (g)
Dinner						
8-oz. (230-g) salmon fillet	420	25	0	46	0	
1½ T. extra-virgin olive oil	170	21	0	0	0	
½ medium tomato, diced	16	0	4	1	2	
½ C. (80 g) spinach (added to the salmon for last 3 minutes of baking)	37	2	3	2	0	
1 C. (225 g) steamed broccoli	34	0	7	2	1	
1 medium sweet potato	103	0	26	2.25	9	
1 T. butter	100	11	1.5	0	1.5	1.5
1 C. (180 g) low-fat (1%) cottage cheese	163	2.25	6	28	6	
with 1 medium peach	38	0.25	9.5	1	8	
16-oz. (480-ml) decaf drink						
Dinner totals	**1,081**	**61.5**	**57**	**82.25**	**27.5**	**1.5**
Evening Snack						
2 C. (300 g) sliced watermelon	92	0	22	2	18	
8-oz. (240-ml) decaf drink						
Snack totals	**92**	**0**	**22**	**2**	**18**	**0**
Day 2 totals	**2,268 cal**	**76.2 g**	**228 g**	**181.25 g**	**119.5 g**	**20.5 g**
		685.8 cal	912 cal	726 cal		
		30%	40%	32%		

					DAY 3	
	Calories	Fat (g)	Carbs (g)	Protein (g)	Sugar (g)	Simple Sugar (g)
Breakfast						
3-egg omelet	220	15	1	20	0	
with ¼ C. (40 g) spinach and ¼ C. (40 g) diced tomato	20	1	3	3	2	
½ slice wholemeal toast	64	1	12	2	1	
1 T. peanut butter	100	8	3	4	1.5	1.5
1 large sliced orange	86	0	22	2	17	

	Calories	Fat (g)	Carbs (g)	Protein (g)	Sugar (g)	Simple Sugar (g)
12-oz. (350-ml) caffeinated or decaf coffee or tea, or water						
Breakfast totals	**490**	**25**	**39**	**31**	**21.5**	**1.5**
Midmorning Snack						
50-g protein shake	200	0	0	50	0	
½ medium banana	50	0	14	0.5	7	7
1 C. (240 ml) skimmed milk (always okay to swap almond milk with skimmed milk anywhere in the plan)	86	0	12	8	12	12
½ C. (70 g) ice (12 oz./350 ml) liquid total in shake)						
Snack totals	**336**	**0**	**26**	**58.5**	**19**	**19**
Lunch						
8-oz. (230-g) salmon fillet OR	415	25	0	45	0	
two 6-oz. (170-g) chicken breasts (The above swap is good anywhere in the plan)	405	8	0	72	0	
2½ C. (100 g) chopped romaine lettuce	15	0	3	1	1	
with 1½ T. extra-virgin olive oil	180	21	0	0	0	
and 1 T. Parmesan cheese	22	1.5	0.2	2	0	
and 10 small black olives	36	3.25	2	0	0	
1 medium apple, sliced	72	0	19	0	14	
16-oz. (480-ml) decaf drink						
Lunch totals	**740**	**41**	**24.2**	**48**	**15**	**0**
Dinner						
8 oz. (230 g) baked scallops	300	7	6	42	0	
over 1 C. (115 g) whole-wheat pasta	174	1	37	7.5	1	
with 1 T. extra-virgin olive oil	120	14	0	0	0	
and 1 C. (240 ml) tomato pasta sauce	185	6	28	5	22	22
16-oz. (480-ml) decaf drink						
Dinner totals	**759**	**28**	**71**	**54.5**	**23**	**22**
Evening Snack						
1 C. (150 g) fresh fruit	46	0	11	1	9	
8-oz. (240-ml) decaf drink						
Snack totals	**46**	**0**	**11**	**1**	**9**	

	Calories	Fat (g)	Carbs (g)	Protein (g)	Sugar (g)	Simple Sugar (g)
Day 3 totals	2,371 cal	94.6 g	171 g	192.5 g	71.5 g	42.5 g
		851.4 cal	684 cal	770 cal		
		36%	29%	32%		

DAY 4

	Calories	Fat (g)	Carbs (g)	Protein (g)	Sugar (g)	Simple Sugar (g)
Breakfast						
60-g protein shake	280	1	7	60	0	
1 T. sugar-free caramel syrup	45	0	12	0	0	
½ medium banana	50	0	14	0.5	7	7
½ C. (120 ml) skimmed milk (always okay to swap almond milk with skimmed milk anywhere in the plan)	43	0	6	4	6	6
½ C. (70 g) ice (12 oz./350 ml liquid total in shake)						
Breakfast totals	**418**	**1**	**39**	**64.5**	**13**	**13**
Midmorning Snack						
1 slice wholemeal toast	128	2	24	4	2	
2 T. peanut butter	200	16	6	8	3	3
8-oz. (240-ml) decaf drink						
Snack totals	**328**	**18**	**30**	**12**	**5**	**3**
Lunch						
8-oz. (230-g) salmon fillet salad	415	25	0	45	0	
with 2½ C. (100 g) romaine lettuce	15	0	3	1	1	
1 T. extra-virgin olive oil	120	14	0	0	0	
Red wine vinegar	0	0	0	0	0	
and 1 T. Parmesan cheese	22	1.5	0.2	2	0	
and 10 small black olives	26	3.25	2	0	0	
1 medium apple	72	0	19	0	14	
16-oz. (480-ml) decaf drink						
Lunch totals	**740**	**44**	**24.2**	**48**	**15**	**0**

	Calories	Fat (g)	Carbs (g)	Protein (g)	Sugar (g)	Simple Sugar (g)
Dinner						
Two 8-oz. (230-g) chicken breasts	472	10	0	85	0	
½ C. (120 g) sundried tomato pesto sauce	200	12	18	4	10	10
1 C. (160 g) chopped peppers	30	0	7	1	4	
1 C. (160 g) spinach, cooked	74	4	7	5	1	
1 T. extra-virgin olive oil	120	14	0	0	0	
6 oz. (170 g) unsweetened Greek yogurt	100	0	7	18	7	7
with ½ medium apple, diced	36	0	9	0	7	
16-oz. (480-ml) decaf drink						
Dinner totals	**900**	**40**	**50**	**113**	**31**	**17**
Evening Snack						
23-g protein bar with <3g sugar	200	6	16	23	3	3
12-oz. (350-ml) decaf drink						
Snack totals	**200**	**6**	**16**	**23**	**3**	**3**
Day 4 totals	**2,526 cal**	**109 g**	**159.2 g**	**261.5 g**	**75 g**	**36 g**
		981 cal	637 cal	1,046 cal		
		39%	24.6%	40%		

DAY 5

	Calories	Fat (g)	Carbs (g)	Protein (g)	Sugar (g)	Simple Sugar (g)
Breakfast						
2-oz. (60 g) fillet steak	123	6	0	11	0	
2 scrambled eggs	144	10	1	12	0	
OR ½ C. (70 g) smoked salmon with 1 t. lemon juice The above swap (salmon swapped with steak and eggs) is good anywhere in the plan	80	3	0	12	0	
½ wholemeal bagel	150	1	30	5	1	
¼ C. (40 g) diced peppers	7	0	2	0	1	
½ C. (80 g) diced tomato	8	0	2	0	1	
1 medium apple, sliced	72	0	19	0	14	

	Calories	Fat (g)	Carbs (g)	Protein (g)	Sugar (g)	Simple Sugar (g)
1 T. peanut butter	100	8	3	4	1.5	1.5
8-oz. (240-ml) caffeinated or decaf coffee or tea, or water						
Breakfast totals	**417**	**12**	**56**	**21**	**18.5**	**1.5**
Midmorning Snack						
20-g protein bar	200	6	16	20	2	2
12-oz. (350-ml) decaf drink						
Snack totals	**200**	**6**	**16**	**20**	**2**	**2**
Lunch						
8-oz. (230-g) turkey burger	440	24	0	50	0	
on wholemeal bun	140	1	27	7	4	
with 1 T. ketchup	15	0	3.5	0.25	3	3
4 sliced dill pickles	32	1	9	0.5	4	
½ C. (60 g) coleslaw	41	2	7.5	1	0	
1 medium peach	38	0.25	9.5	1	8	
12-oz. (350-ml) decaf drink						
Lunch totals	**706**	**28.25**	**56.5**	**59.75**	**19**	**3**
Dinner						
2 small veal chops	406	22	0	48	0	
1 T. barbecue sauce	70	0	17	0	16	16
1 C. (200 g) grilled veggies	25	0	4	2	1	
2 T. extra-virgin olive oil	240	28	0	0	0	
16-oz. (480-ml) decaf drink						
Dinner totals	**740**	**50**	**21**	**50**	**17**	**16**
Evening Snack						
1 C. (225 g) unsweetened Greek yogurt	130	0	9	23	9	9
¼ C. (30 g) sliced strawberries	20	0	5	0	4	
Mix with 5 g protein powder	20	0	0	5	0	
12-oz. (350-ml) decaf drink						
Snack totals	**170**	**0**	**14**	**28**	**13**	**9**
Day 5 totals	**2,233 cal**	**96 g**	**163 g**	**184 g**	**69.5 g**	**31.5 g**
		866 cal	648 cal	736 cal		
		38%	29%	33%		

DAY 6

	Calories	Fat (g)	Carbs (g)	Protein (g)	Sugar (g)	Simple Sugar (g)
Breakfast						
60-g protein shake	280	1	7	60	0	
1 T. sugar-free caramel syrup	45	0	12	0	0	
½ medium banana	50	0	14	0.5	7	7
½ C. (120 ml) skimmed milk (always okay to swap almond milk with skimmed milk anywhere in the plan)	43	0	6	4	6	6
½ C. (70 g) ice (12 oz./350 ml liquid total in shake)						
Breakfast totals	**428**	**1**	**39**	**64.5**	**13**	**13**
Midmorning Snack						
1 slice wholemeal toast	128	2	24	4	2	
2 T. peanut butter	200	16	6	8	3	3
8-oz. (240-ml) decaf drink						
Snack totals	**328**	**18**	**30**	**12**	**5**	**3**
Lunch						
8-oz. (230-g) fillet steak salad OR	480	22	0	44	0	
8-oz. (230-g) salmon fillet salad The above swap is good anywhere in the plan, served or prepared with the following ingredients:	415	25	0	45	0	
2½ C. (100 g) romaine lettuce	15	0	3	1	1	
with 1½ T. extra-virgin olive oil	180	21	0	0	0	
and red wine vinegar	0	0	0	0	0	
and 1 T. Parmesan cheese	22	1.5	0.2	2	0	
and 10 small black olives	26	3.25	2	0	0	
1 medium apple	72	0	19	0	14	
16-oz. (480-ml) decaf drink						
Lunch totals	**740**	**51**	**24.2**	**48**	**15**	**0**
Dinner						
Two 8-oz. (230-g) chicken breasts	472	10	0	85	0	
½ C. (120 g) sundried tomato pesto sauce	200	12	18	4	10	10

	Calories	Fat (g)	Carbs (g)	Protein (g)	Sugar (g)	Simple Sugar (g)
1 C. (160 g) chopped peppers	30	0	7	1	4	
1 C. (160 g) spinach, steamed	74	4	7	5	1	
1 T. extra-virgin olive oil	120	14	0	0	0	
1 C. (225 g) unsweetened Greek yogurt	130	0	9	23	9	9
with ½ medium apple, diced	36	0	9	0	7	
16-oz. (480-ml) decaf drink						
Dinner totals	**930**	**42**	**50**	**118**	**31**	**19**
Evening Snack						
23-g protein bar	200	6	16	23	3	3
12-oz. (350-ml) decaf drink						
Snack totals	**200**	**6**	**16**	**23**	**3**	**3**
Day 6 totals	**2,626 cal**	**118 g**	**159.2 g**	**265.5 g**	**67 g**	**36 g**
		1,062 cal	636 cal	1,062 cal		
		40%	24%	40%		

DAY 7

	Calories	Fat (g)	Carbs (g)	Protein (g)	Sugar (g)	Simple Sugar (g)
Breakfast						
25-g protein shake	100	0	0	25	0	
½ C. (70 g) ice (12 oz./350 ml liquid total in shake)						
½ medium banana	55	0	14	1	7	7
½ C. (120 ml) skimmed milk (always okay to swap almond milk with skimmed milk anywhere in the plan)	43	0	6	4	6	6
1 T. peanut butter	100	8	3	4	1.5	1.5
Breakfast totals	**298**	**8**	**22**	**34**	**14.5**	**14.5**
Midmorning Snack						
1 medium peach	38	0.25	9	1	8	
¼ C. (30 g) almonds	206	18	7	7.5	1.5	
8-oz. (240-ml) decaf drink						
Snack totals	**244**	**18.25**	**16**	**8.5**	**9.5**	**0**

	Calories	Fat (g)	Carbs (g)	Protein (g)	Sugar (g)	Simple Sugar (g)
Lunch						
Roast beef sandwich (6 thin slices)	336	20	0	33	0	
2 slices wholemeal bread	256	4	48	8	4	
1 T. mustard	9	0.5	1	0.6	0.5	0.5
7 wholemeal pita crisps	110	3	18	4	0.5	
16-oz. (480-ml) decaf drink						
Lunch totals	**711**	**27.5**	**67**	**45.6**	**5**	**0.5**
Dinner						
8 oz. (230 g) baked scallops	300	7	6	42	0	
⅓ C. (20 g) sundried tomatoes	46	5	10	2.5	7	
1 T. extra-virgin olive oil	119	14	0	0	0	
1 C. (130 g) brown rice, cooked	215	2	44	5	1	
mixed with 1 C. (225 g) broccoli	34	0	7	2	1	
½ C. (40 g) romaine lettuce	15	0	3	1	1	
with 3 T. balsamic vinaigrette	38	1.5	6	0	4	4
and 10 small black olives	36	3.2	5	2	0	0
1 C. (225 g) unsweetened Greek yogurt	130	0	9	23	9	9
OR ½ C. (90 g) low-fat (1%) cottage cheese	81	1	3	14	3	3
The above swap (½ C./90 g cottage cheese for yogurt) is good anywhere in the plan						
with ½ C. (60 g) strawberries	27	0.25	7	0.5	4	
16-oz. (480-ml) decaf drink						
Dinner totals	**959**	**33.5**	**94**	**76**	**29**	**16**
Evening Snack						
Five 7-inch (18-cm) celery stalks	30	0.3	7	1	1	
2 T. peanut butter	200	16	6	8	3	3
8-oz. (240-ml) decaf drink						
Snack totals	**230**	**16.3**	**13**	**9**	**4**	**3**
Day 7 totals	**2,442 cal**	**103 g**	**213 g**	**173 g**	**62 g**	**31 g**
		927 cal	952 cal	692 cal		
		38%	38%	28%		

Phase 1/Week 2 Shopping List

8 ounces (230 grams) smoked salmon

Lemons for lemon juice (they should be left over from Week 1)

English muffins (they should be left over from Week 1)

8 ounces (230 grams) ground lean steak for burger

Two small lamb chops

Fat-free unsweetened Greek yogurt

Ingredients for whole-grain pancake mix (recipe on page 264)

8 ounces (230 grams) minced lean turkey for turkey burger

Two 8-ounce (230-gram) salmon fillets

Four 8-ounce (230-gram) skinless chicken breasts

One can sundried tomato pesto sauce (low-sugar)

One bag wholemeal pita crisps

Ingredients for avocado tuna salad (recipe on page 262)

Eighteen slices deli roast beef or turkey (swap any time)

8 ounces (230 grams) fresh scallops

⅓ C. (20 grams) sundried tomatoes

Bottle of low-fat balsamic vinaigrette

40-gram pre-made protein shake (such as Muscle Milk)

8 ounces (230 grams) sugar-free ice cream

One small carton of low-sugar instant porridge

One medium sweet potato

Phase 1/Week 2 Daily Menus

						DAY 8
	Calories	Fat (g)	Carbs (g)	Protein (g)	Sugar (g)	Simple Sugar (g)
Breakfast						
½ C. (70 g) smoked salmon with 1 t. lemon juice	80	3	0	12	0	
½ wholemeal bagel	150	1	30	5	1	
OR 1 wholemeal English muffin The above swap is good anywhere in the plan	129	1	26	5	1	
¼ C. (40 g) diced peppers	7	0	2	0	1	
½ C. (80 g) diced tomato	8	0	2	0	1	
1 medium apple, sliced	72	0	19	0	14	
1 T. peanut butter	100	8	3	4	1.5	1.5
8-oz. (240-ml) caffeinated or decaf coffee or tea, or water						
Breakfast totals	**417**	**12**	**56**	**21**	**18.5**	**1.5**

	Calories	Fat (g)	Carbs (g)	Protein (g)	Sugar (g)	Simple Sugar (g)
Midmorning Snack						
20-g protein bar (<2g sugar)	200	6	16	20	2	2
12-oz. (350-ml) drink						
Snack totals	**200**	**6**	**16**	**20**	**2**	**2**
Lunch						
8-oz. (230-g) turkey burger	440	24	0	50	0	
on wholemeal bun	140	1	27	7	4	
with 1 T. ketchup	15	0	3.5	0.25	3	3
4 sliced dill pickles	32	1	9	0.5	4	
½ C. (60 g) coleslaw	41	2	7.5	1	3	3
1 medium peach	38	0.25	9.5	1	8	
12-oz. (350-ml) drink						
Lunch totals	**706**	**28.25**	**56.5**	**59.75**	**19**	**6**
Dinner						
2 small veal chops	406	22	0	48	0	
2 T. Joe's Tgio sauce	22	0	4	1	3	3
1 C. (200 g) grilled veggies	25	0	4	2	1	
2 T. extra-virgin olive oil	240	28	0	0	0	
16-oz. (480-ml) decaf drink						
Dinner totals	**693**	**50**	**8**	**51**	**4**	**3**
Evening Snack						
1 C. (225 g) unsweetened Greek yogurt	130	0	9	23	9	9
¼ C. (30 g) sliced strawberries	15	0	4	0	3	
mixed with 5 g protein powder	20	0	0	5	0	
12-oz. (350-ml) decaf drink						
Snack totals	**165**	**0**	**13**	**28**	**12**	**9**
Day 8 totals	**2,181 cal**	**96 g**	**149 g**	**179.5 g**	**55.5 g**	**21.5 g**
		866 cal	600 cal	718 cal		
		37%	27.5%	33%		

DAY 9

	Calories	Fat (g)	Carbs (g)	Protein (g)	Sugar (g)	Simple Sugar (g)
Breakfast						
½ C. (70 g) smoked salmon with 1 t. lemon juice	80	3	0	12	0	
½ wholemeal bagel	50	1	26	5	1	
1 medium apple, sliced	72	0	19	0	14	
1 T. peanut butter	100	8	3	4	1.5	1.5
8-oz. (240-ml) caffeinated or decaf coffee or tea, or water						
Breakfast totals	**402**	**12**	**48**	**21**	**16.5**	**1.5**
Midmorning Snack						
20-g protein bar	200	6	16	20	2	2
12-oz. (350-ml) drink						
Snack totals	**200**	**6**	**16**	**20**	**2**	**2**
Lunch						
8-oz. (230-g) steak burger	560	45	0	40	0	
1 wholemeal bun	140	1	27	7	4	
with 1 T. ketchup	15	0	3.5	0.25	3	3
4 sliced dill pickles	32	1	9	0.5	4	
½ C. (65 g) brown rice, cooked	108	0.5	22	5	0	
with 1 t. butter	33	3.5	0	0	0	
1 medium peach	38	0.25	9.5	1	8	
12-oz. (350-ml) drink						
Lunch totals	**926**	**52**	**70**	**54.5**	**19**	**3**
Dinner						
2 small lamb chops, grilled and seasoned to taste	224	11	0	32	0	
with 1 T. barbecue sauce	70	0	17	0	16	16
1 C. (200 g) grilled veggies	25	0	4	2	1	
2 T. extra-virgin olive oil	240	28	0	0	0	
16-oz. (480-ml) decaf drink						
Dinner totals	**559**	**39**	**23**	**34**	**17**	**16**

	Calories	Fat (g)	Carbs (g)	Protein (g)	Sugar (g)	Simple Sugar (g)
Evening Snack						
½ C. (60 g) sliced strawberries	40	0	10	0	8	
1 T. fat-free unsweetened Greek yogurt	20	1	3	0	0	
mixed with 5 g protein powder	20	0	0	5	0	
12-oz. (350-ml) decaf drink						
Snack totals	**80**	**1**	**13**	**5**	**8**	**0**
Day 9 totals	**2,167 cal**	**110 g**	**170 g**	**130 g**	**62.5 g**	**22.5 g**
		990 cal	680 cal	520 cal		
		45%	31%	24%		

DAY 10

	Calories	Fat (g)	Carbs (g)	Protein (g)	Sugar (g)	Simple Sugar (g)
Breakfast						
2 whole-grain pancakes	160	4	30	3.5	7	
with ½ C. (60 g) blueberries	83	0	21	1	14	
and 4 T. sugar-free maple syrup	10	0	4	0	0	
1 C. (100 g) grapes	110	0	29	1	25	
12-oz. (350-ml) caffeinated or decaf coffee or tea, or water						
Breakfast totals	**363**	**4**	**84**	**5.5**	**46**	**0**
Midmorning Snack						
50-g protein shake	200	0	0	50	0	
2 T. sugar-free strawberry syrup	10	0	4	0	0	
with ½ medium banana	50	0	14	0.5	7	7
½ C. (120 ml) skimmed milk (always okay to swap almond milk with skimmed milk anywhere in the plan)	43	0	6	4	6	6
(12 oz./350 ml liquid total in shake)						
Snack totals	**303**	**0**	**24**	**50.5**	**13**	**13**

	Calories	Fat (g)	Carbs (g)	Protein (g)	Sugar (g)	Simple Sugar (g)
Lunch						
1 C. (200 g) tuna salad	383	10	3	30	2	2
½ avocado	160	15	9	2	0	
1 sliced medium tomato	22	0	5	1	3	
4 whole-wheat crackers	72	3	10	1.5	0	
16-oz. (480-ml) decaf drink						
Lunch totals	**637**	**28**	**27**	**34.5**	**5**	**2**
Dinner						
Two 8-oz. (230-g) chicken breasts	472	10	0	88	0	
½ C. (120 g) sundried tomato pesto	200	12	18	4	10	10
1 C. (160 g) chopped peppers	30	0	7	1	4	
1 C. (160 g) spinach, cooked	74	4	7	5	1	
1 T. extra-virgin olive oil	120	14	0	0	0	
1 C. (225 g) unsweetened Greek yogurt	130	0	9	23	9	9
with ½ medium apple, sliced	36	0	9	0	7	
16-oz. (480-ml) decaf drink						
Dinner totals	**1,062**	**40**	**50**	**121**	**31**	**19**
Evening Snack						
2 C. (300 g) diced watermelon	92	0	22	2	18	
8-oz. (240-ml) decaf drink						
Snack totals	**92**	**0**	**22**	**2**	**18**	**0**
Day 10 totals	**2,457 cal**	**72.3 g**	**214 g**	**217 g**	**113 g**	**34 g**
		651 cal	856 cal	868 cal		
		26%	34%	35%		

DAY 11

	Calories	Fat (g)	Carbs (g)	Protein (g)	Sugar (g)	Simple Sugar (g)
Breakfast						
25-g protein shake	100	0	0	25	0	
½ medium banana	52	0	13	1	7	7
½ C. (120 ml) skimmed milk (always okay to swap almond milk with skimmed milk anywhere in the plan)	43	0	6	4	6	6

	Calories	Fat (g)	Carbs (g)	Protein (g)	Sugar (g)	Simple Sugar (g)
1 T. peanut butter	100	8	3	4	1.5	1.5
½ C. (70 g) ice (12 oz./350 ml liquid total in shake)						
Breakfast totals	**295**	**8**	**22**	**34**	**14.5**	**14.5**
Midmorning Snack						
1 medium peach	38	0.25	9	1	8	
¼ C. (30 g) almonds	206	18	7	7.5	1.5	
8-oz. (240-ml) decaf drink						
Snack totals	**244**	**18.25**	**16**	**8.5**	**9.5**	**0**
Lunch						
Roast beef or turkey sandwich (6 thin slices) Swap roast beef for turkey anywhere in the plan	336	20	0	33	0	
2 slices wholemeal bread	256	4	48	8	4	
1 T. mustard	9	0.5	1	0.6	0.5	0.5
7 wholemeal pita crisps	110	3	18	4	0.5	
16-oz. (480-ml) decaf drink						
Lunch totals	**711**	**27.5**	**67**	**45.6**	**5**	**0.5**
Dinner						
8 oz. (230 g) baked scallops	300	7	6	42	0	
⅓ C. (20 g) sundried tomatoes	46	5	10	2.5	7	
1 T. extra-virgin olive oil	119	14	0	0	0	
1 C. (130 g) brown rice, cooked	215	2	44	5	1	
mixed with 1 C. (225 g) broccoli	34	0	7	2	1	
2½ C. (100 g) romaine lettuce	15	0	3	1	1	
with 3 T. balsamic vinaigrette	38	1.5	6	0	4	4
and 10 small black olives	36	3.25	2	0	0	
½ C. (60 g) strawberries	27	0.25	7	0.5	4	
16-oz. (480-ml) decaf drink						
Dinner totals	**829**	**33.5**	**85**	**53**	**18**	**4**
Evening Snack						
Five 7-inch (18-cm) celery stalks	30	0.3	7	1	1	
2 T. peanut butter	200	16	6	8	3	3

	Calories	Fat (g)	Carbs (g)	Protein (g)	Sugar (g)	Simple Sugar (g)
8-oz. (240-ml) decaf drink						
Snack totals	230	16.3	13	9	4	3
Day 11 totals	2,309 cal	103 g	203 g	150 g	80 g	22 g
		932 cal	812 cal	600 cal		
		40%	35%	26%		

DAY 12

	Calories	Fat (g)	Carbs (g)	Protein (g)	Sugar (g)	Simple Sugar (g)
Breakfast						
40-g pre-made protein shake (14 oz./400 ml liquid total in shake)	220	3	7	40	2	2
Breakfast totals	220	3	7	40	2	2
Midmorning Snack						
1 medium peach	38	0.25	9	1	8	
¼ C. (30 g) almonds	206	18	7	7.5	1.5	
8-oz. (240-ml) decaf drink						
Snack totals	244	18.25	16	8.5	9.5	0
Lunch						
Roast beef sandwich (6 thin slices)	336	20	0	33	0	
2 slices wholemeal bread	256	4	48	8	4	
1 T. mustard	9	0.5	1	0.6	0.5	0.5
7 wholemeal pita crisps	110	3	18	4	0.5	
16-oz. (480-ml) decaf drink						
Lunch totals	711	27.5	67	45.6	5	0.5
Dinner						
8 oz. (230 g) baked scallops	300	7	6	42	0	
⅓ C. (20 g) sundried tomatoes	46	5	10	2.5	7	
1 T. extra-virgin olive oil	119	14	0	0	0	
½ C. (65 g) brown rice, cooked	107	1	22	3	1	
mixed with 1 C. (225 g) broccoli	34	0	7	2	1	
2½ C. (100 g) romaine lettuce	15	0	3	1	1	

	Calories	Fat (g)	Carbs (g)	Protein (g)	Sugar (g)	Simple Sugar (g)
with 3 T. balsamic vinaigrette	38	1.5	6	0	4	4
and 10 small black olives	36	3.25	2	0	0	
½ C. (60 g) strawberries	27	0.25	7	0.5	4	
16-oz. (480-ml) decaf drink						
Dinner totals	**722**	**31.5**	**61**	**53**	**18**	**4**
Evening Snack						
Five 7-inch (18-cm) celery stalks	30	0.3	7	1	1	
2 T. peanut butter	200	16	6	8	3	3
8-oz. (240-ml) decaf drink						
Snack totals	**230**	**16.3**	**13**	**9**	**4**	**3**
Day 12 totals	**2,127 cal**	**100 g**	**166 g**	**156 g**	**38.5 g**	**9.5 g**
		900 cal	752 cal	624 cal		
		41%	33%	29%		

DAY 13

	Calories	Fat (g)	Carbs (g)	Protein (g)	Sugar (g)	Simple Sugar (g)
Breakfast						
2 hard-boiled eggs	155	10	1	12	1	
1 slice wholemeal toast	128	2	23	4	2	
1 T. peanut butter	100	8	3	4	1.5	1.5
12-oz. (350-ml) caffeinated or decaf coffee or tea, or water						
Breakfast totals	**383**	**20**	**27**	**20**	**4.5**	**1.5**
Midmorning Snack						
1 large orange	86	0	22	2	17	
8-oz. (240-ml) sugar-free drink						
Snack totals	**86**	**0**	**22**	**2**	**17**	**0**
Lunch						
Roast beef sandwich (6 thin slices)	336	20	0	33	0	
2 slices wholemeal bread	256	4	48	8	4	
1 T. mustard	9	0.5	1	0.6	0.5	0.5

	Calories	Fat (g)	Carbs (g)	Protein (g)	Sugar (g)	Simple Sugar (g)
7 wholemeal pita crisps	110	3	18	4	0.5	
16-oz. (480-ml) decaf drink						
Lunch totals	**711**	**27.5**	**67**	**45.6**	**5**	**0.5**
Dinner						
8 oz. (230 g) sautéed/steamed prawns	323	5	3	62	0	
⅓ C. (20 g) sundried tomatoes	46	5	10	2.5	7	
1 T. extra-virgin olive oil	119	14	0	0	0	
1 C. (130 g) brown rice, cooked	215	2	44	5	1	
mixed with 1 C. (225 g) broccoli	34	0	7	2	1	
2½ C. (100 g) romaine lettuce	15	0	3	1	1	
with 3 T. balsamic vinaigrette	38	1.5	6	0	4	4
and 10 small black olives	36	3.25	2	0	0	
½ C. (120 ml) sugar-free vanilla ice cream	110	6	16	2	4	4
with ½ C. (60 g) strawberries	27	0.25	7	0.5	4	
16-oz. (480-ml) decaf drink						
Dinner totals	**964**	**38**	**94**	**75**	**18**	**8**
Evening Snack						
1 C. (240 ml) sugar-free applesauce with ½ t. cinnamon	50	0	12	0	11 (yes!)	11
8-oz. (240-ml) decaf drink						
Snack totals	**50**	**0**	**12**	**0**	**11**	**11**
Day 13 totals	**2,194 cal**	**85.5 g**	**222 g**	**150 g**	**59.5 g**	**21 g**
		765.5 cal	888 cal	570 cal		
		35%	40%	26%		

DAY 14						
	Calories	Fat (g)	Carbs (g)	Protein (g)	Sugar (g)	Simple Sugar (g)
Breakfast						
1 C. (240 ml) reduced-sugar instant porridge	145	2	25	6	2	
1 medium banana	105	0	27	1	14	

	Calories	Fat (g)	Carbs (g)	Protein (g)	Sugar (g)	Simple Sugar (g)
½ C. (120 ml) skimmed milk (always okay to swap almond milk with skimmed milk anywhere in the plan	43	0	6	4	6	6
1 medium orange	62	0	15	1	12	
12-oz. (350-ml) caffeinated or decaf coffee or tea, or water						
Breakfast totals	**355**	**2**	**73**	**12**	**34**	**6**
Midmorning Snack						
50-g protein shake	200	0	0	50	0	
1 C. (240 ml) skimmed milk (always okay to swap almond milk with skimmed milk anywhere in the plan)	86	0	12	8	12	12
½ C. (60 g) strawberries	26	0	7	0.5	4	
¼ C. (35 g) ice						
12-oz. (350-ml) decaf drink						
Snack totals	**312**	**0**	**19**	**58.5**	**16**	**12**
Lunch						
1 C. (225 g) turkey chili	256	8	22	25	5	5
made with ⅛ C. (20 g) spinach	7	0	1	1	0	
1 T. Parmesan cheese	22	1.4	0	0.2	0	
4 whole-wheat crackers	76	3	11	1.5	0	
1 C. (100 g) grapes	110	0.3	29	1	25	
16-oz. (480-ml) decaf drink						
Lunch totals	**471**	**12.7**	**63**	**28.7**	**30**	**5**
Dinner						
8-oz. (230-g) salmon fillet	420	25	0	46	0	
1½ T. extra-virgin olive oil	170	21	0	0	0	
and red wine vinegar, to taste	0	0	0	0	0	
½ medium tomato, diced	16	0	4	1	2	
½ C. (80 g) spinach (added to the salmon for the last 3 minutes of baking)	37	2	3	2	0	
1 C. (225 g) steamed broccoli	34	0	7	2	1	
1 medium sweet potato	103	0	26	2.25	3	3
1 T. butter	100	11	0	0	0	

	Calories	Fat (g)	Carbs (g)	Protein (g)	Sugar (g)	Simple Sugar (g)
1 C. (180 g) low-fat (1%) cottage cheese	163	2.25	6	28	6	
with 1 medium peach	38	0.25	9.5	1	8	
16-oz. (480-ml) decaf drink						
Dinner totals	**1,081**	**61.5**	**55.5**	**82.25**	**20**	**3**
Evening Snack						
2 C. (300 g) sliced watermelon	92	0	22	2	18	
8-oz. (240-ml) decaf drink						
Snack totals	**92**	**0**	**22**	**2**	**18**	
Day 14 totals	**2,311 cal**	**76.2 g**	**213.5 g**	**182.5 g**	**124 g**	**20 g**
		685.8 cal	854 cal	730 cal		
		30%	37%	32%		

Phase 2/Week 3 Shopping List

Ingredients for whole-grain pancake mix (recipe on page 264)

Ingredients for avocado tuna salad (recipe on page 262) (can swap tuna with chicken, salmon, or steak)

Two 8-ounce (230-gram) chicken breasts

One can sundried tomato pesto sauce (low-sugar)

Fresh spinach

Fresh peppers

Six medium apples

Unsweetened Greek yogurt or low-fat cottage cheese

One dozen medium eggs

4 ounces (115 grams) thinly sliced low-fat mozzarella cheese

Four slices deli turkey breast

Wholemeal bread

Three fresh tomatoes

Assorted fresh raw veggies

Low-fat mayonnaise

8-ounce (230-gram) tuna steak

8 ounces (230 grams) low-fat lemon dill sauce

Twelve fresh asparagus spears

8 ounces (230 grams) minced turkey

One small bag reduced-fat crisps

One 8-ounce (230-gram) and one 4-ounce (115-gram) fillet steak

12 ounces (340 grams) cooked shrimp

Two medium baking potatoes

Fresh mushrooms

Fresh blueberries and strawberries

Fresh cantaloupe melon

Four bananas

Four turkey rashers

Two 8-ounce (230-gram) tilapia fillets

Ingredients for chili (recipe on page 256)

1 C. (200 grams) cooked corn—fresh (preferred) or canned

One large orange

4-ounce (115-gram) and 8-ounce (230-gram) veggie burger

One head lettuce

Fresh grapes

25-gram and 40-gram pre-made protein shake (such as Muscle Milk)

8 ounces (230 grams) smoked salmon

Phase 2/Week 3 Daily Menus

DAY 15

	Calories	Fat (g)	Carbs (g)	Protein (g)	Sugar (g)	Simple Sugar (g)
Breakfast (Treat Meal)*						
2 whole-grain pancakes	160	4	30	3.5	7	
with ½ C. (60 g) blueberries	83	0	21	1	14	
4 T. sugar-free maple syrup	10	0	4	0	0	
1 C. (100 g) grapes	110	0	29	1	25	
12-oz. (350-ml) caffeinated or decaf coffee or tea, or water						
Breakfast totals	**363**	**4**	**84**	**5.5**	**46**	**0**
Midmorning Snack						
1 medium apple, sliced	72	0	19	0	14	
¼ C. (30 g) almonds	206	18	7	8	2	
8-oz. (240-ml) decaf drink						
Snack totals	**278**	**18**	**26**	**8**	**16**	**0**
Lunch						
1 C. (200 g) tuna salad	383	10	3	30	2	2
½ avocado	160	15	9	2	0	
1 sliced medium tomato	22	0	5	1	3	
4 whole-wheat crackers	72	3	10	1.5	0	
16-oz. (480-ml) decaf drink						
Lunch totals	**637**	**28**	**27**	**34.5**	**5**	**2**
Dinner						
Two 8-oz. (320-g) chicken breasts	472	10	0	88	0	
½ C. (120 g) sundried tomato pesto	200	12	18	4	10	
1 C. (160 g) chopped peppers	30	0	7	1	4	
1 C. (160 g) spinach, cooked	74	4	7	5	1	
1 T. extra-virgin olive oil	120	14	0	0	0	
6 oz. (170 g) unsweetened Greek yogurt	100	0	9	23	6	6
with ½ sliced medium apple	36	0	9	0	7	
16-oz. (480-ml) decaf drink						
Dinner totals	**1,032**	**40**	**50**	**121**	**28**	**6**

	Calories	Fat (g)	Carbs (g)	Protein (g)	Sugar (g)	Simple Sugar (g)
Evening Snack						
2 medium apples	144	0	42	2	28	
2 T. peanut butter	200	16	6	8	3	3
8-oz. (240-ml) decaf drink						
Snack totals	**344**	**16**	**48**	**10**	**31**	**3**
Day 15 totals	**2,654 cal**	**106 g**	**234 g**	**178 g**	**126 g**	**11 g**
		954 cal	936 cal	712 cal		
		36%	35%	27%		

*Remember that "Treat Meals" are the meals in each phase where I went a little wild and gave you some extra treats. Don't swap these meals, or you might end up getting too many calories by the end of the week.

DAY 16

	Calories	Fat (g)	Carbs (g)	Protein (g)	Sugar (g)	Simple Sugar (g)
Breakfast						
3-egg omelet	220	15	1	20	0	
½ C. (80 g) diced tomato	16	0	3	1	2.5	
½ C. (80 g) spinach	37	2	4	3	0	
1 slice mozzarella cheese	86	5.5	1	7	0	
1 C. (150 g) assorted fruit	80	0	20	1	14	
12-oz. (350-ml) caffeinated or decaf coffee or tea, or water						
Breakfast totals	**439**	**22.5**	**29**	**32**	**17**	**0**
Midmorning Snack						
¼ C. (30 g) almonds	206	18	7	8	2	
1 medium banana	105	0	27	1	14	
8-oz. (240-ml) drink						
Snack totals	**311**	**18**	**34**	**9**	**16**	**0**
Lunch						
Turkey sandwich (4 slices)	120	2	4	20	4	
2 slices wholemeal bread	256	4	48	8	4	
2 slices medium tomato	7	0	2	0	1	
1 T. low-fat mayo	49	5	1	0	1	1

	Calories	Fat (g)	Carbs (g)	Protein (g)	Sugar (g)	Simple Sugar (g)
1 C. (150 g) raw veggies	25	0.25	6	1	3	
16-oz. (480-ml) decaf drink						
Lunch totals	**457**	**11.25**	**61**	**29**	**13**	**1**
Dinner						
8-oz. (230-g) tuna steak	180	2	0	40	0	
with 1 T. low-fat lemon dill sauce	130	6	6	1	2	2
6 spears asparagus	18	0	6	2	0	
1 T. extra-virgin olive oil	120	14	0	0	0	
2½ C. (100 g) romaine lettuce	15	0	3	1	1	
with 1½ T. balsamic vinaigrette	38	1.5	6	0	2	2
and 10 small black olives	36	3	2	0	0	
1 C. (160 g) sliced strawberries	53	0.5	13	1	8	
1 T. unsweetened Greek yogurt	25	1.5	2	0	1	1
16-oz. (480-ml) decaf drink						
Dinner totals	**615**	**33.5**	**38**	**45**	**18**	**5**
Evening Snack						
50-g protein shake	200	0	0	50	0	
½ medium banana	52	0	14	0.5	5	5
2 T. sugar-free chocolate syrup (8 oz./240 ml liquid total in shake)	15	0	5	1	0	
Snack totals	**267**	**0**	**19**	**51.5**	**7**	**5**
Day 16 totals	**2,089 cal**	**86 g**	**181 g**	**167 g**	**72 g**	**11 g**
		774 cal	724 cal	668 cal		
		37%	34%	31%		

DAY 17

	Calories	Fat (g)	Carbs (g)	Protein (g)	Sugar (g)	Simple Sugar (g)
Breakfast						
3 hard- or soft-boiled eggs	220	15	1	20	0	
1 slice wholemeal toast	128	2	24	4	2	
1 C. (120 g) strawberries	53	0.5	13	1	8	

	Calories	Fat (g)	Carbs (g)	Protein (g)	Sugar (g)	Simple Sugar (g)
12-oz. (350-ml) caffeinated or decaf coffee or tea, or water						
Breakfast totals	**401**	**17.5**	**38**	**25**	**10**	**0**
Midmorning Snack						
23-g protein bar	200	6	16	23	3	3
8-oz. (240-ml) decaf drink						
Snack totals	**200**	**6**	**16**	**23**	**3**	**3**
Lunch						
8-oz. (230-g) turkey burger	440	24	0	50	0	
1 wholemeal bun	140	1	27	7	4	
1 T. ketchup	15	0	3.5	0.25	3	3
4 dill pickle slices	0	0	0	0	0	
1 C. (30 g) reduced-fat potato crisps	94	4	13	1.5	0	
1 medium apple	72	0	19	0	14	
16-oz. (480-ml) decaf drink						
Lunch totals	**761**	**29**	**62.5**	**59**	**21**	**3**
Dinner						
8-oz. (230-g) fillet steak	480	22	0	44	0	
4 oz. (115 g) cooked prawns	80	1	0	18	0	
2 T. extra-virgin olive oil	240	28	0	0	0	
1 medium baked potato	121	0	28	3	2	2
1 t. butter	32	2.5	1	1.5	0.5	
½ C. (45 g) mushrooms	7.5	0	1	1	0.5	
1 C. (160 g) spinach with garlic seasoning, cooked	74	4	7	5	1	
½ C. (60 g) blueberries/raspberries	83	0	21	1	14	
16-oz. (480-ml) decaf drink						
Dinner totals	**1,117.5**	**57.5**	**58**	**73.5**	**18**	**2**
Evening Snack						
6 oz. (170 g) unsweetened Greek yogurt	100	0	9	23	6	6
¼ C. (30 g) strawberries	15	0	4	0	3	
12-oz. (350-ml) decaf drink						
Snack totals	**115**	**0**	**13**	**23**	**9**	**6**

	Calories	Fat (g)	Carbs (g)	Protein (g)	Sugar (g)	Simple Sugar (g)
Day 17 totals	2,594 cal	110 g	187.5 g	203.5 g	61 g	14 g
		990 cal	750 cal	814 cal		
		37%	28%	31%		

DAY 18

	Calories	Fat (g)	Carbs (g)	Protein (g)	Sugar (g)	Simple Sugar (g)
Breakfast (Treat Meal)*						
½ C. (75 g) cantaloupe melon balls	30	0	8	0.5	7	
½ medium apple, sliced	36	0	9	0	7	
½ medium banana	53	0	13	0.5	7	
1 T. peanut butter	94	8	3	4	1.5	1.5
4 turkey rashers	244	16	0	20	0	
½ slice wholemeal toast	64	1	12	2	1	
12-oz. (350-ml) caffeinated or decaf coffee or tea, or water						
Breakfast totals	**521**	**25**	**45**	**27**	**23.5**	**1.5**
Midmorning Snack						
¼ C. (40 g) pistachios	175	14	8	7	2.5	
12-oz. (350-ml) decaf drink						
Snack totals	**175**	**14**	**8**	**7**	**2.5**	**0**
Lunch						
Tilapia salad with 2½ C. (100 g) romaine lettuce	15	0	3	1	1	
8 oz. (230 g) tilapia fillet	186	2	0	42	0	
3 T. balsamic vinaigrette	38	1.5	6	0	4	4
5 small black olives	18	1.5	1	0	0	
½ C. (80 g) diced tomato	8	0	2	0	1	
2 sliced hard-boiled eggs	144	10	1	12	0	
16-oz. (480-ml) decaf drink						
Lunch totals	**409**	**15**	**13**	**55**	**6**	**4**
Dinner						
2 C. (450 g) chili with lean minced beef	512	16	44	50	5	5
1 medium baked potato	121	0	28	3	2	

	Calories	Fat (g)	Carbs (g)	Protein (g)	Sugar (g)	Simple Sugar (g)
(with 1 T. butter)	100	11	0	0	0	
½ C. (50 g) canned corn	60	1	11	2	7	
16-oz. (480-ml) decaf drink						
Dinner totals	**793**	**28**	**83**	**55**	**14**	**5**
Evening Snack						
20-g protein bar	200	6	16	20	2	2
½ C. (50 g) grapes	55	0	14.5	0.5	12.5	
8-oz. (240-ml) decaf drink						
Snack totals	**255**	**6**	**30.5**	**20.5**	**14.5**	**2**
Day 18 totals	**2,153 cal**	**88 g**	**178.5 g**	**164.5 g**	**62.5 g**	**12.5 g**
		792 cal	**714 cal**	**658 cal**		
		37%	**33%**	**30%**		

*Remember that "Treat Meals" are the meals in each phase where I went a little wild and gave you some extra treats. Don't swap these meals, or you might end up getting too many calories by the end of the week.

DAY 19

	Calories	Fat (g)	Carbs (g)	Protein (g)	Sugar (g)	Simple Sugar (g)
Breakfast						
3 scrambled eggs	220	15	1	20	0	
1 slice wholemeal toast	128	2	24	4	2	
1 medium orange	85	0	21	1	17	
12-oz. (350-ml) caffeinated or decaf coffee or tea, or water						
Breakfast totals	**433**	**17**	**46**	**25**	**19**	**0**
Midmorning Snack						
40-g pre-made protein shake (total 14 oz./400 ml liquid)	220	3	7	40	2	2
Snack totals	**220**	**3**	**7**	**40**	**2**	**2**
Lunch						
1 C. (200 g) chicken/turkey/tuna salad sandwich	383	10	3	30	2	2
2 slices wholemeal bread	256	4	48	8	4	
2 slices medium tomato	7	0	2	0	1	

	Calories	Fat (g)	Carbs (g)	Protein (g)	Sugar (g)	Simple Sugar (g)
1 medium apple	72	0	18	0	14	
OR						
2 C. (300 g) diced watermelon	86	0	21.5	1.5	16	
16-oz. (480-ml) decaf coffee, tea, or water						
Lunch totals	**732**	**14**	**96.5**	**39.5**	**23**	**2**
Dinner						
8 oz. (230 g) sautéed/steamed/ baked prawns	241	4	2	46	0	
(use no more than 1 T. olive oil)	120	14	0	0	0	
1 medium baked potato	120	0	28	3	2	2
(with 1 T. butter)	100	11	0	0	0	
6 medium asparagus spears	18	0	6	2	0	
(with 1 T. butter)	100	11	0	0	0	
16-oz. (480-ml) decaf coffee, tea, or water						
Dinner totals	**699**	**40**	**36**	**51**	**2**	**2**
Evening Snack						
2 medium apples	144	0	42	2	28	
2 T. peanut butter	200	16	6	8	3	3
8-oz. (240-ml) decaf coffee, tea, or water						
Snack totals	**344**	**16**	**48**	**10**	**31**	**3**
Day 19 totals	**2,428 cal**	**84 g**	**224.5 g**	**185.5 g**	**68 g**	**9 g**
		756 cal	898 cal	742 cal		
		31%	37%	31%		

DAY 20

	Calories	Fat (g)	Carbs (g)	Protein (g)	Sugar (g)	Simple Sugar (g)
Breakfast						
4-oz. (115 g) fillet steak	240	11	0	22	0	
2 scrambled eggs	144	10	1	12	0	
1 slice wholemeal toast	128	2	24	4	2	

	Calories	Fat (g)	Carbs (g)	Protein (g)	Sugar (g)	Simple Sugar (g)
5 oz. (145 g) unsweetened Greek yogurt	80	0	0	15	5	5
1 large orange	86	0	22	2	17	
12-oz. (350-ml) caffeinated or decaf coffee or tea, or water						
Breakfast totals	**678**	**23**	**47**	**55**	**25**	**5**
Midmorning Snack						
¼ C. (30 g) almonds	206	18	7	8	2	
12 oz. (350 ml) water						
Snack totals	**206**	**18**	**7**	**8**	**2**	**0**
Lunch						
4-oz. (115-g) veggie burger	201	7	16	19	1	
Lettuce wrap	0	0	0	0	0	
1 t. ketchup	5	0	1	0	1	1
2 medium apples	144	0	38	0	28	
16-oz. (480-ml) decaf iced tea or water						
Lunch totals	**350**	**7**	**55**	**19**	**30**	**1**
Dinner						
Two 4-oz. (115-g) tilapia fillets	186	2	0	42	0	
2 C. (320 g) spinach, cooked	148	8	14	10	2	
1 medium baked potato	121	0	28	3	2	2
with 1 T. regular sour cream	27	3	0	0	0	
1 C. (100 g) grapes	110	0	29	1	25	
16-oz. (480-ml) decaf iced tea or water						
Dinner totals	**592**	**13**	**71**	**56**	**29**	**2**
Evening Snack						
40-g pre-made protein shake (total 14 oz./400 ml liquid)	220	3	7	40	2	2
Snack totals	**220**	**3**	**7**	**40**	**2**	**2**
Day 20 totals	**2,046 cal**	**64 g**	**187 g**	**178 g**	**88 g**	**10 g**
		576 cal	748 cal	712 cal		
		28%	37%	35%		

DAY 21

	Calories	Fat (g)	Carbs (g)	Protein (g)	Sugar (g)	Simple Sugar (g)
Breakfast						
1 C. smoked salmon (140 g) with 1 t. lemon juice	160	6	0	24	0	
½ wholemeal bagel	150	1	30	5	1	
¼ C. (30 g) diced orange	7	0	2	0	1	
½ C. (80 g) diced tomato	8	0	2	0	1	
1 medium banana	105	0	27	1	14	
12-oz. (350-ml) caffeinated or decaf coffee or tea, or water						
Breakfast totals	**430**	**7**	**61**	**30**	**17**	**0**
Midmorning Snack						
25-g protein Muscle Milk shake	220	9	10	25	3	3
8-oz. (240-ml) decaf drink						
Snack totals	**220**	**9**	**10**	**25**	**3**	**3**
Lunch						
1½ C. (300 g) tuna salad	550	40	4.5	45	2	2
½ avocado	160	15	9	2	0	
1 medium tomato, sliced	22	0	5	1	3	
4 whole-wheat crackers	72	3	10	1.5	0	
16-oz. (480-ml) decaf drink						
Lunch totals	**804**	**58**	**28.5**	**49.5**	**5**	**2**
Dinner						
8-oz. (230 g) veggie burger	402	14	32	38	2	
1 wholemeal bun	140	1	27	7	4	
1 T. ketchup	15	0	3.5	0.25	3	3
4 slices dill pickles	0	0	0	0	0	
½ C. (65 g) brown rice, cooked	107	1	22	2.5	0.5	
16-oz. (480-ml) decaf drink						
Dinner totals	**664**	**16**	**84.5**	**48**	**9.5**	**3**
Evening Snack						
¼ C. (30 g) almonds	206	18	7	8	2	
12-oz. (350-ml) decaf drink						
Snack totals	**206**	**18**	**7**	**8**	**2**	**0**

	Calories	Fat (g)	Carbs (g)	Protein (g)	Sugar (g)	Simple Sugar (g)
Day 21 totals	2,324 cal	108 g	181 g	161 g	34.5 g	8 g
		945 cal	724 cal	634 cal		
		41%	31%	27%		

Phase 2/Week 4 Shopping List

2 ounces (60 grams) smoked salmon

Wholemeal bagel or wholemeal English muffin

Three red peppers

Cantaloupe or honeydew melon

8 ounces (230 grams) lean minced turkey

Dill pickles

Three medium peaches

½ cup (60 grams) no-sugar coleslaw

Two small veal chops

Assorted veggies for grilling

1 C. (200 grams) brown rice

Unsweetened Greek yogurt or low-fat cottage cheese

One dozen medium eggs

Low-fat turkey sausage

Wholemeal bread

Four medium oranges

Pistachio nuts

Five 23-gram protein bars (such as Pure Protein brand)

One package tomato basil tortilla wraps

Six slices low-fat deli roast beef or turkey

Fresh grapes

Wholemeal pita crisps

Dijon mustard

8-ounce (230-gram) cod fillet

Three fresh tomatoes

8 ounces (230 grams) fresh broccoli

Two medium sweet potatoes

Butter

Fresh strawberries

Sugar-free ice cream

Whole-grain cereal

Six medium bananas

Fresh blueberries

Four slices low-fat deli turkey breast

½ loaf rye bread (or substitute with wholemeal bread)

4-ounce (115-gram) fillet steak

Two medium white baking potatoes

Six asparagus spears

8-ounce (230-gram) tilapia fillet

Fresh spinach

Cinnamon

Protein powder (such as Isopure)

Skimmed milk

Sugar-free almond milk

Natural peanut butter

Three 40-gram pre-made protein shakes (such as Muscle Milk)

4-ounce (115-gram) veggie burger

Lettuce

Four medium apples

8-ounce (230-gram) salmon fillet

Parmesan cheese

One can small black olives

Fresh berries (1 cup/125 grams)

Whole-grain pancake mix (recipe on page 264)

Sugar-free maple syrup

Four turkey rashers

Ingredients for avocado tuna salad (recipe on page 262); also for swaps with chicken, turkey, or steak)

One avocado

Whole-wheat crackers

8-ounce (230-gram) snapper fillet

Lemon pepper

Fresh mushrooms

Fresh raspberries

Two garlic cloves or garlic salt seasoning

1-pound (450-gram) bag almonds

8 ounces (230 grams) skinless chicken breast for chicken salad (recipe on page 255)

Romaine lettuce

Balsamic vinaigrette or red wine vinegar

8 ounces (230 grams) scallops

1 can sundried tomatoes

Extra-virgin olive oil

Brown rice

Soy sauce

Smoked salmon for salmon sushi (recipe on page 266)

One package of at least ten cherry tomatoes (these are great to munch on at any time)

Romaine lettuce and rocket mix

8-ounce (230-gram) tuna steak

One bottle low-fat lemon dill sauce

Phase 2/Week 4 Daily Menus

DAY 22

Breakfast	Calories	Fat (g)	Carbs (g)	Protein (g)	Sugar (g)	Simple Sugar (g)
2 oz. (60 g) smoked salmon	66	2.5	0	10.5	0	
½ wholemeal bagel	150	1	30	5	1	
1 t. lemon juice	3	0	1	0	0.3	0.3
¼ C. (40 g) diced peppers	10	0	2	0.4	1.5	
1 medium sliced apple	72	0	19	0	14	
with 1 T. peanut butter	100	8	3	4	1.5	1.5
12-oz. (350-ml) caffeinated or decaf coffee or tea, or water						
Breakfast totals	**401**	**11.5**	**55**	**20**	**18.3**	**1.8**
Midmorning Snack						
½ C. (75 g) cantaloupe or honeydew melon balls	30	0	8	0.5	7	
12-oz. (350-ml) sugar-free drink						
Snack totals	**30**	**0**	**8**	**0.5**	**7**	**0**
Lunch						
8-oz. (230-g) turkey burger (no bun)	440	24	0	50	0	
1 T. ketchup	15	0	3.5	0.25	3	3
4 slices dill pickles	0	0	0	0	0	
½ C. (60 g) coleslaw	41	1.5	7.5	1	0	
1 medium peach	38	2.5	9.5	1	8	
8-oz. (240-ml) sugar-free drink						
Lunch totals	**534**	**26**	**20.5**	**52.25**	**11**	**3**
Dinner						
2 small veal chops	406	22	0	48	0	
1 C. (200 g) grilled veggies	147	4	23	5	5	
2 T. extra-virgin olive oil	240	28	0	0	0	
1 C. (130 g) brown rice, cooked	107	1	22	2.5	0.5	
12-oz. (350-ml) sugar-free drink						
Dinner totals	**900**	**57**	**45**	**55**	**5.5**	**0**

	Calories	Fat (g)	Carbs (g)	Protein (g)	Sugar (g)	Simple Sugar (g)
Evening Snack						
6 oz. (170 g) unsweetened Greek yogurt	100	0	8	18	7	7
12-oz. (350-ml) sugar-free drink						
Snack totals	**100**	**0**	**8**	**18**	**7**	**7**
Day 22 totals	1,965 cal	94.5 g	136.5 g	146 g	37.5 g	11.8 g
		850.5 cal	546 cal	584 cal		
		43%	28%	30%		

DAY 23

	Calories	Fat (g)	Carbs (g)	Protein (g)	Sugar (g)	Simple Sugar (g)
Breakfast						
3 hard-boiled eggs	220	15	1	20	0	
2 links turkey sausage	60	3.5	1	8	0	
½ slice wholemeal toast	64	1	12	4	1	
with ½ t. butter	15	6	0	0	0	
1 medium orange	85	0	21	1	14	
16-oz. (480-ml) caffeinated or decaf coffee or tea, or water						
Breakfast totals	**429**	**19.5**	**35**	**33**	**15**	**0**
Midmorning Snack						
¼ C. (40 g) pistachios	175	14	8	7	2.5	
23-g protein bar	200	6	16	23	3	3
12-oz. (350-ml) drink						
Snack totals	**375**	**20**	**24**	**30**	**5.5**	**3**
Lunch						
Roast beef wrap (6 slices)	336	20	0	33	0	
Tomato basil tortilla wrap	210	4.5	35	6	4	4
1 T. Dijon mustard	4	0	0.5	0.25	0	
1 slice cheddar cheese	70	6	0	4	0	
7 wholemeal pita crisps	110	3	18	4	0.5	0.5

	Calories	Fat (g)	Carbs (g)	Protein (g)	Sugar (g)	Simple Sugar (g)
1 C. (100 g) grapes	110	0	29	1	25	
12-oz. (350-ml) sugar-free drink						
Lunch totals	**840**	**15.5**	**82.5**	**48.25**	**29**	**4.5**
Dinner						
8-oz. (230-g) cod fillet	160	2	0	30	0	
grilled with ¼ C. (40 g) diced tomato	4	0	1	0	0	
1 T. extra-virgin olive oil	119	14	0	0	0	
1 C. (225 g) steamed broccoli	34	0	7	2	1	
½ medium sweet potato	50	0	11	1	4	4
1 t. butter	30	2	0	0	0	
16-oz. (480-ml) sugar-free drink						
Dinner totals	**397**	**18**	**19**	**33**	**5**	**4**
Evening Snack						
½ C. (60 g) strawberries	27	0.25	7	0.5	0.4	
with 2 t. sugar-free ice cream	50	1	5	0	0	
⅕ scoop (10 g) protein powder	40	0	0	10	0	
8-oz. (240-ml) sugar-free drink						
Snack totals	**77**	**1.25**	**12**	**10.5**	**0**	**0**
Day 23 totals	**2,118 cal**	**74.5 g**	**176.5 g**	**155 g**	**58 g**	**11.5 g**
		670.5 cal	706 cal	620 cal		
		32%	33%	30%		

DAY 24

	Calories	Fat (g)	Carbs (g)	Protein (g)	Sugar (g)	Simple Sugar (g)
Breakfast (Treat Meal)*						
1 C. (30 g) whole-grain cereal	125	0	26	3	5	
¼ C. (60 ml) skimmed milk (always okay to swap almond milk with skimmed milk anywhere in the plan)	21	0	3	2	3	3
½ medium banana	50	0	13	1	7	
¼ C. (30 g) blueberries	41	0	10	0.5	7	

	Calories	Fat (g)	Carbs (g)	Protein (g)	Sugar (g)	Simple Sugar (g)
16-oz. (480-ml) caffeinated or decaf coffee or tea, or water						
Breakfast totals	**237**	**0**	**52**	**6.5**	**23**	**3**
Midmorning Snack						
4 slices turkey breast	90	2	4	15	3	
1 slice rye bread	83	1	15	3	1	1
with light glaze of Dijon mustard	2	0	0	0	0	
12-oz. (350-ml) sugar-free drink						
Snack totals	**175**	**3**	**19**	**18**	**4**	**1**
Lunch						
4-oz. (115-g) grilled fillet steak	240	11	0	22	0	
with 1 T. extra virgin olive oil	119	14	0	0	0	
1 medium baked potato	120	0	28	3	1	1
½ C. (60 g) grilled asparagus	13	0	2	1.5	1	
12-oz. (350-ml) sugar-free drink						
Lunch totals	**493**	**25**	**30**	**25**	**1**	**1**
Dinner						
8-oz. (230-g) grilled tilapia fillet seasoned with garlic salt and cinnamon	220	4	0	45.5	0	
in 2 T. extra-virgin olive oil	240	28	0	0	0	
2 C. (320 g) steamed spinach	14	0.25	2	2	0.25	
½ medium baked sweet potato	51	0	12	1.5	3	3
with 1 T. butter	100	11	1.5	0	1.5	1.5
½ C. (60 g) strawberries	26	0	7	0.5	4	
12-oz. (350-ml) sugar-free drink						
Dinner totals	**650**	**39.25**	**22.5**	**49.5**	**8.75**	**4.5**
Evening Snack						
60-g protein shake	280	1	7	60	2	2
1 T. sugar-free caramel syrup	45	0	12	0	0	
¼ C. (60 ml) skimmed milk (always okay to swap almond milk with skimmed milk anywhere in the plan)	21	0	3	2	3	3

	Calories	Fat (g)	Carbs (g)	Protein (g)	Sugar (g)	Simple Sugar (g)
¼ C. (60 ml) almond milk	10	0	0.3	0.4	0	
1 C. (140 g) ice	0	0	0	0	0	
Snack totals	356	1	22.3	62.4	5	5
Day 24 totals	1,911 cal	71.25 g	146 g	151.4 g	43 g	14.5 g
		641 cal	584 cal	605 cal		
		34%	31%	32%		

*Remember that "Treat Meals" are the meals in each phase where I went a little wild and gave you some extra treats. Don't swap these meals, or you might end up getting too many calories by the end of the week.

DAY 25

	Calories	Fat (g)	Carbs (g)	Protein (g)	Sugar (g)	Simple Sugar (g)
Breakfast						
3-egg omelet	220	15	1	20	0	
with ¼ C. (40 g) spinach and ¼ C. (40 g) diced tomato	20	1	3	3	2	
½ slice wholemeal toast	64	1	12	2	1	
1 T. peanut butter	100	8	3	4	1.5	1.5
1 large sliced orange	86	0	22	2	17	
12-oz. (350-ml) caffeinated or decaf coffee or tea, or water						
Breakfast totals	490	25	39	31	21.5	1.5
Midmorning Snack						
40-g pre-made protein shake (14 oz./400 ml liquid total in shake)	220	3	7	40	2	2
Snack totals	220	3	7	40	2	2
Lunch						
4-oz. (115-g) veggie burger	201	7	16	19	1	
wrapped in lettuce	0	0	0	0	0	
1 slice tomato	4	0	1	0	0.5	
2 medium apples	144	0	38	0	28	
16-oz. (480-ml) sugar-free drink						
Lunch totals	349	7	55	19	28	0

	Calories	Fat (g)	Carbs (g)	Protein (g)	Sugar (g)	Simple Sugar (g)
Dinner						
8-oz. (230-g) salmon fillet	415	25	0	45	0	
2½ C. (100 g) romaine lettuce	15	0	3	1	1	
with 1½ T. extra-virgin olive oil	180	21	0	0	0	
and 1 T. Parmesan cheese	22	1.5	0.2	2	0	
and 10 small black olives	36	3.25	2	0	0	
16-oz. (480-ml) decaf drink						
Dinner totals	**668**	**51**	**5.2**	**47**	**1**	**0**
Evening Snack						
1 C. (125 g) mixed fresh berries	70	0	17	2	12	
40-g pre-made protein shake	220	3	7	40	2	2
8-oz. (240-ml) sugar-free drink						
Snack totals	**290**	**3**	**24**	**42**	**14**	**2**
Day 25 totals	**2,017 cal**	**89 g**	**130 g**	**179 g**	**66 g**	**5.5 g**
		800 cal	**521 cal**	**716 cal**		
		39%	**28%**	**35%**		

DAY 26

	Calories	Fat (g)	Carbs (g)	Protein (g)	Sugar (g)	Simple Sugar (g)
Breakfast (Treat Meal)*						
2 whole-grain pancakes (include 20 g. sugar-free protein powder in the batter)	240	4	30	23.5	7	
with ½ C. (60 g) blueberries	83	0	21	1	14	
4 T. sugar-free maple syrup	10	0	4	0	0	
6 turkey rashers	183	13	2	15	0	
12-oz. (350-ml) caffeinated or decaf coffee or tea, or water						
Breakfast totals	**516**	**17**	**57**	**39.5**	**21**	**0**
Midmorning Snack						
2 sliced hard-boiled eggs	144	10	1	12	0	
12-oz. (350-ml) sugar-free drink						
Snack totals	**144**	**10**	**1**	**12**	**0**	**0**

	Calories	Fat (g)	Carbs (g)	Protein (g)	Sugar (g)	Simple Sugar (g)
Lunch						
1 C. (200 g) tuna salad (with 2 T. low-fat mayo)	383	10	14.5	30	2	2
½ avocado	160	15	9	2	0	
1 medium tomato, sliced	22	0	5	1	3	
4 whole-wheat crackers	72	3	10	1.5	0	
16-oz. (480-ml) decaf drink						
Lunch totals	**637**	**28**	**38.5**	**34.5**	**5**	**2**
Dinner						
8-oz. (230-g) snapper fillet grilled with lemon pepper	227	3	0	46.5	0	
and 2 T. extra-virgin olive oil	240	28	0	0	0	
1 medium baked potato	121	0	28	3	2	2
1 t. butter	32	2.5	1	1.5	0.5	0.5
½ C. (90 g) mushrooms	7.5	0	1	1	0.5	
1 C. (160 g) spinach with garlic, cooked	74	4	7	5	1	
½ C. (160 g) blueberries or raspberries	83	0	21	1	14	
16-oz. (480-ml) decaf drink						
Dinner totals	**784.5**	**37.5**	**58**	**58**	**18**	**2.5**
Evening Snack						
23-g protein bar	200	6	16	23	3	3
12-oz. (350-ml) decaf drink						
Snack totals	**200**	**6**	**16**	**23**	**3**	**3**
Day 26 totals	**2,281 cal**	**98.5 g**	**170.5 g**	**167 g**	**47 g**	**7.5 g**
		886.5 cal	682 cal	668 cal		
		39%	30%	29%		

*Remember that "Treat Meals" are the meals in each phase where I went a little wild and gave you some extra treats. Don't swap these meals, or you might end up getting too many calories by the end of the week.

DAY 27

	Calories	Fat (g)	Carbs (g)	Protein (g)	Sugar (g)	Simple Sugar (g)
Breakfast						
3 poached eggs	220	15	1	20	0	
1 slice wholemeal toast	128	2	24	4	2	
1 C. (120 g) strawberries	53	0.5	13	1	8	
12-oz. (350-ml) caffeinated or decaf coffee or tea, or water						
Breakfast totals	**401**	**17.5**	**38**	**25**	**10**	**0**
Midmorning Snack						
¼ C. (30 g) almonds	206	18	7	8	2	
1 medium banana	105	0	27	1	14	
8-oz. (240-ml) drink						
Snack totals	**311**	**18**	**34**	**9**	**16**	**0**
Lunch						
Chicken salad with 8-oz. (230-g) skinless grilled chicken breast	281	11	0	42	0	
and 2½ C. (100 g) romaine lettuce	15	0	3	1	1	
and 3 T. balsamic vinaigrette	38	1.5	6	0	4	
and 5 small black olives	18	1.5	1	0	0	
and ½ C. (80 g) diced tomato	8	0	2	0	1	
and 2 sliced hard-boiled eggs	144	10	1	12	0	
16-oz. (480-ml) decaf drink						
Lunch totals	**505**	**24**	**13**	**55**	**6**	**0**
Dinner						
8 oz. (230 g) baked scallops	300	7	6	42	0	
⅓ C. (20 g) sundried tomatoes	46	5	10	2.5	7	3
1 T. extra-virgin olive oil	119	14	0	0	0	
1 C. (130 g) brown rice, cooked	215	2	44	5	1	
mixed with 1 C. (225 g) steamed broccoli	34	0	7	2	1	
12-oz. (350-ml) sugar-free drink						
Dinner totals	**763**	**28**	**67**	**51.5**	**9**	**3**

	Calories	Fat (g)	Carbs (g)	Protein (g)	Sugar (g)	Simple Sugar (g)
Evening Snack						
1 C. (120 g) mixed fresh berries	70	0	17	2	12	
8-oz. (240-ml) decaf drink						
Snack totals	**70**	**0**	**17**	**2**	**12**	**0**
Day 27 totals	2,050 cal	87.5 g	169 g	143 g	53 g	3 g
		783.5 cal	676 cal	572 cal		
		38%	33%	28%		

DAY 28

	Calories	Fat (g)	Carbs (g)	Protein (g)	Sugar (g)	Simple Sugar (g)
Breakfast						
3-egg omelet	220	15	1	20	0	
with ¼ C. (40 g) spinach and ¼ C. (40 g) diced tomato	20	1	3	3	2	
½ slice wholemeal toast	64	1	12	2	1	
1 T. peanut butter	100	8	3	4	1.5	1.5
1 large sliced orange	86	0	22	2	17	
12-oz. (350-ml) caffeinated or decaf coffee or tea, or water						
Breakfast totals	**490**	**25**	**39**	**31**	**21.5**	**1.5**
Midmorning Snack						
40-g pre-made protein shake	220	3	7	40	2	2
Snack totals	**220**	**3**	**7**	**40**	**2**	**2**
Lunch						
6 oz. (170 g) smoked salmon (for salmon sushi)	396	15	0	63	0	
stuffed with ½ C. (65 g) brown rice, cooked	108	0.5	22	5	0	
2 C. (80 g) romaine lettuce and rocket mix	12	0	2	1	1	
with 5 cherry tomatoes	15	0	3	1	2	
and 5 black olives	18	1.5	1	0	0	
2 T. soy sauce	20	0	0	2	1	1
12-oz. (350-ml) sugar-free drink						
Lunch totals	**569**	**17**	**28**	**72**	**4**	**1**

	Calories	Fat (g)	Carbs (g)	Protein (g)	Sugar (g)	Simple Sugar (g)
Dinner						
8-oz. (230-g) tuna steak	180	2	0	40	0	
with 2 T. low-fat lemon dill sauce	130	11	6	1	4	4
6 spears asparagus	18	0	6	2	0	
1 T. extra-virgin olive oil	120	14	0	0	0	
1 C. (160 g) sliced strawberries	53	0.5	13	1	8	
1 T. unsweetened Greek yogurt	25	1.5	2	0	1	1
16-oz. (480-ml) sugar-free drink						
Dinner totals	**526**	**29**	**27**	**44**	**13**	**5**
Evening Snack						
¼ C. (30 g) almonds	206	18	7	8	2	
12-oz. (350-ml) decaf drink						
Snack totals	**206**	**18**	**7**	**8**	**2**	**0**
Day 28 totals	**2,011 cal**	**92 g**	**108 g**	**195 g**	**42.5 g**	**9.5 g**
		828 cal	432 cal	780 cal		
		41%	22%	38%		

Phase 3/Week 5 Shopping List

One dozen medium eggs
Wholemeal bread
Butter
Extra-virgin olive oil
Two 23-gram protein bars (such as Pure Protein brand)
8 ounces (230 grams) lean minced turkey
Dill pickles (sliced)
Ketchup
Reduced-fat potato crisps
Four medium apples
Two 4-ounce (115-gram) and one 6-ounce (170-gram) fillet steak
4 ounces (115 grams) prawns
Five medium baking potatoes
Fresh mushrooms
Fresh strawberries, raspberries, and blueberries
Cantaloupe or honeydew melon
Natural peanut butter
Four turkey rashers
Six medium bananas

Eight medium apples
Three 40-gram pre-made protein shakes (such as Muscle Milk)
Fresh grapes
Ingredients for turkey chili (recipe on page 256)
Fresh spinach
Whole-wheat crackers
Parmesan cheese
Two 8-ounce (230-grams) skinless chicken breasts
Sundried tomato pesto sauce (low-sugar)
Three red peppers
8 ounces (230 grams) unsweetened fat-free Greek yogurt
8 ounce (230 gram) bag almonds
Three medium to large oranges
Two 4-ounce (115-gram) veggie burgers
Two 4-ounce (115-gram) tilapia fillets

Sour cream
Mozzarella cheese
Assorted fresh fruit
Eight slices deli turkey
Low-fat mayonnaise
Assorted raw veggies
Two 8-ounce (230-gram) tuna steaks
Low-fat lemon dill sauce
Fresh asparagus spears
Romaine and butterhead lettuce
Balsamic vinaigrette
1 can black olives
Protein powder (such as Isopure brand)
Sugar-free chocolate syrup
Whole-grain pancake mix (recipe on page 264)
Sugar-free maple syrup
8-ounce (230-gram) snapper fillet
Lemon pepper

Phase 3/Week 5 Daily Menus

DAY 29

	Calories	Fat (g)	Carbs (g)	Protein (g)	Sugar (g)	Simple Sugar (g)
Breakfast						
3 hard- or soft-boiled eggs	220	15	1	20	0	
1 slice wholemeal toast	128	2	24	4	2	
1 C. (120 g) strawberries	53	0.5	13	1	8	
12-oz. (350-ml) caffeinated or decaf coffee or tea, or water						
Breakfast totals	**401**	**17.5**	**38**	**25**	**10**	**0**

	Calories	Fat (g)	Carbs (g)	Protein (g)	Sugar (g)	Simple Sugar (g)
Midmorning Snack						
23-g protein bar	200	6	16	23	3	3
8-oz. (240-ml) decaf drink						
Snack totals	**200**	**6**	**16**	**23**	**3**	**3**
Lunch						
8-oz. (230-g) turkey burger	440	24	0	50	0	
1 T. ketchup	15	0	3.5	0.25	3	3
4 slices dill pickle	0	0	0	0	0	
1 C. (30 g) reduced-fat potato crisps	94	4	13	1.5	0	
1 medium apple	72	0	19	0	14	
16-oz. (480-ml) decaf drink						
Lunch totals	**620**	**28**	**35.5**	**52**	**17**	**3**
Dinner						
4-oz. (115-g) fillet steak	240	11	0	22	0	
4 oz. (115 g) cooked prawns	80	1	0	18	0	
2 T. extra-virgin olive oil	240	28	0	0	0	
1 medium baked potato	121	0	28	3	2	2
1 t. butter	32	2.5	1	1.5	0.5	0.5
½ C. (90 g) mushrooms	7.5	0	1	1	0.5	
1 C. (160 g) spinach with garlic, cooked	74	4	7	5	1	
½ C. (60 g) blueberries/raspberries	83	0	21	1	14	
16-oz. (480-ml) sugar-free drink						
Dinner totals	**877.5**	**46.5**	**58**	**51.5**	**18**	**2.5**
No Snack						
Day 29 totals	**2,098.5 cal**	**97 g**	**147 g**	**151.5 g**	**48 g**	**8.5 g**
		872 cal	588 cal	604 g		
		41%	28%	30%		

DAY 30

	Calories	Fat (g)	Carbs (g)	Protein (g)	Sugar (g)	Simple Sugar (g)
Breakfast (Treat Meal)*						
½ C. (75 g) cantaloupe melon balls	30	0	8	0.5	7	
½ medium apple, sliced	36	0	9	0	7	
½ medium banana	53	0	13	0.5	7	
1 T. peanut butter	94	8	3	4	1.5	1.5
4 turkey rashers	122	9	0	9.5	0	
½ slice wholemeal toast	64	1	12	2	1	
12-oz. (350-ml) caffeinated or decaf coffee or tea, or water						
Breakfast totals	**399**	**18**	**45**	**16.5**	**23.5**	**1.5**
Midmorning Snack						
40-g pre-made protein shake	220	3	7	40	2	2
Snack totals	**220**	**3**	**7**	**40**	**2**	**2**
Lunch						
1 C. (225 g) beef or turkey chili	256	8	22	25	5	5
made with ⅛ C. (20 g) spinach	7	0	1	1	0	
1 T. Parmesan cheese	22	1.4	0	2	0	
4 whole-wheat crackers	76	3	11	1.5	0	
1 C. (100 g) grapes	110	0.3	29	1	25	
16-oz. (480-ml) sugar-free drink						
Lunch totals	**471**	**12.7**	**63**	**30.5**	**25**	**5**
Dinner						
Two 8-oz. (230-g) chicken breasts	472	10	0	88	0	
¼ C. (60 g) sundried tomato pesto	100	6	9	2	5	5
1 C. (160 g) chopped peppers	30	0	7	1	4	
1 C. (160 g) spinach, cooked	74	4	7	5	1	
1 T. extra-virgin olive oil	120	14	0	0	0	
½ medium apple, sliced	36	0	9	0	7	
16-oz. (480-ml) decaf drink						
Dinner totals	**832**	**28**	**32**	**96**	**17**	**5**
No Snack						
12-oz. (350-ml) sugar-free drink						

	Calories	Fat (g)	Carbs (g)	Protein (g)	Sugar (g)	Simple Sugar (g)
Day 30 totals	1,922 cal	62 g	147 g	182 g	72 g	13.5 g
		560 cal	588 cal	728 cal		
		30%	31%	38%		

*Remember that "Treat Meals" are the meals in each phase where I went a little wild and gave you some extra treats. Don't swap these meals, or you might end up getting too many calories by the end of the week.

DAY 31

	Calories	Fat (g)	Carbs (g)	Protein (g)	Sugar (g)	Simple Sugar (g)
Breakfast						
4-oz. (115-g) fillet steak	240	11	0	22	0	
2 scrambled eggs	144	10	1	12	0	
1 slice wholemeal toast	128	2	24	4	2	
5 oz. (145 g) unsweetened Greek yogurt	80	0	0	15	5	5
1 large orange	86	0	22	2	17	
12-oz. (350-ml) caffeinated or decaf coffee or tea, or water						
Breakfast totals	678	23	47	55	25	5
Midmorning Snack						
¼ C. (30 g) almonds	206	18	7	8	2	
12 oz. (350 ml) water						
Snack totals	206	18	7	8	2	0
Lunch						
4-oz. (115-g) veggie burger	201	7	16	19	1	
2 medium apples	144	0	38	0	28	
16-oz. (480-ml) decaf iced tea or water						
Lunch totals	345	7	54	19	29	0
Dinner						
Two 4-oz. (115-g) tilapia fillets	186	2	0	42	0	
2 C. (320 g) spinach, cooked	148	8	14	10	2	
1 medium baked potato	121	0	28	3	2	2
with 1 T. regular sour cream	27	3	0	0	0	
1 C. (100 g) grapes	110	0	29	1	25	

	Calories	Fat (g)	Carbs (g)	Protein (g)	Sugar (g)	Simple Sugar (g)
16-oz. (480-ml) decaf iced tea or water						
Dinner totals	**592**	**13**	**71**	**56**	**29**	**2**
Evening Snack						
40-g pre-made protein shake (total 14 oz./400 ml liquid)	220	3	7	40	2	2
Snack totals	**220**	**3**	**7**	**40**	**2**	**2**
Day 31 totals	**2,041 cal**	**64 g**	**186 g**	**178 g**	**87 g**	**9 g**
		576 cal	744 cal	712 cal		
		28%	36%	35%		

DAY 32

	Calories	Fat (g)	Carbs (g)	Protein (g)	Sugar (g)	Simple Sugar (g)
Breakfast						
3-egg omelet	220	15	1	20	0	
½ C. (80 g) diced tomato	16	0	3	1	2.5	
½ C. (80 g) spinach	37	2	4	3	0	
1 slice mozzarella cheese	86	5.5	1	7	0	
1 C. (150 g) assorted fruit	80	0	20	1	14	
12-oz. (350-ml) caffeinated or decaf coffee or tea, or water						
Breakfast totals	**439**	**22.5**	**29**	**32**	**16.5**	**0**
Midmorning Snack						
¼ C. (30 g) almonds	206	18	7	8	2	
1 medium banana	105	0	27	1	14	
8-oz. (240-ml) drink						
Snack totals	**311**	**18**	**34**	**9**	**16**	**0**
Lunch						
Turkey sandwich (4 slices)	120	2	4	20	4	
2 slices wholemeal bread	256	4	48	8	4	
2 slices medium tomato	7	0	2	0	1	
1 T. low-fat mayo	49	5	1	0	1	1
1 C. (150 g) raw veggies	25	0.25	6	1	3	

	Calories	Fat (g)	Carbs (g)	Protein (g)	Sugar (g)	Simple Sugar (g)
16-oz. (480-ml) decaf drink						
Lunch totals	**457**	**11.25**	**61**	**29**	**13**	**1**
Dinner						
8-oz. (230-g) tuna steak	180	2	0	40	0	
with 1 T. low-fat lemon dill sauce	130	6	6	1	2	2
6 spears asparagus	18	0	6	2	0	
1 T. extra-virgin olive oil	120	14	0	0	0	
2½ C. (100 g) romaine lettuce	15	0	3	1	1	
with 1½ T. balsamic vinaigrette	38	1.5	6	0	2	2
and 10 small black olives	36	3	2	0	0	
1 C. (120 g) sliced strawberries	53	0.5	13	1	8	
1 T. unsweetened Greek yogurt	25	1.5	2	0	1	1
16-oz. (480-ml) decaf drink						
Dinner totals	**615**	**33.5**	**38**	**45**	**18**	**5**
Evening Snack						
50-g protein shake	200	0	0	50	0	
½ medium banana	52	0	14	0.5	5	5
2 T. sugar-free chocolate syrup (8 oz./240 ml liquid total in shake)	15	0	5	1	0	
Snack totals	**267**	**0**	**19**	**51.5**	**7**	**5**
Day 32 totals	**2,089 cal**	**86 g**	**181 g**	**167 g**	**72 g**	**11 g**
		774 cal	724 cal	668 cal		
		37%	34%	31%		

DAY 33

	Calories	Fat (g)	Carbs (g)	Protein (g)	Sugar (g)	Simple Sugar (g)
Breakfast (Treat Meal)*						
2 whole-grain pancakes	160	4	30	3.5	7	
mixed with 20 g protein powder	80	0	0	20	0	
with ½ C. (60 g) blueberries	83	0	21	1	14	
4 T. sugar-free maple syrup	10	0	4	0	0	
1 medium orange	62	0	15	1	12	

	Calories	Fat (g)	Carbs (g)	Protein (g)	Sugar (g)	Simple Sugar (g)
12-oz. (350-ml) caffeinated or decaf coffee or tea, or water						
Breakfast totals	**395**	**4**	**70**	**25.5**	**33**	**0**
Midmorning Snack						
¼ C. (30 g) almonds	206	18	7	8	2	
12-oz. (350-ml) sugar-free drink						
Snack totals	**206**	**18**	**7**	**8**	**2**	**0**
Lunch						
6-oz. (170-g) fillet steak grilled	360	14	0	30	0	
with 1 T. extra virgin olive oil	119	14	0	0	0	
1 medium baked potato	120	0	28	3	1	1
½ C. (60 g) grilled asparagus	13	0	2	1.5	1	
12-oz. (350-ml) sugar-free drink						
Lunch totals	**612**	**28**	**30**	**34.5**	**2**	**1**
Dinner						
8-oz. (230-g) snapper fillet grilled with lemon pepper	227	3	0	46.5	0	
and 2 T. extra-virgin olive oil	240	28	0	0	0	
1 medium baked potato	121	0	28	3	2	2
1 t. butter	32	2.5	1	1.5	0.5	0.5
½ C. (90 g) mushrooms	7.5	0	1	1	0.5	
1 C. (160 g) spinach with garlic, cooked	74	4	7	5	1	
½ C. (60 g) blueberries/raspberries	83	0	21	1	14	
16-oz. (480-ml) decaf drink						
Dinner totals	**784.5**	**37.5**	**58**	**58**	**18**	**2.5**
Evening Snack						
23-g protein bar	200	6	16	23	3	3
12-oz. (350-ml) decaf drink						
Snack totals	**200**	**6**	**16**	**23**	**3**	**3**
Day 33 totals	**2,197.5 cal**	**93 g**	**181 g**	**149 g**	**58 g**	**3.5**
		837 cal	724 cal	596 cal		
		38%	33%	27%		

*Remember that "Treat Meals" are the meals in each phase where I went a little wild and gave you some extra treats. Don't swap these meals, or you might end up getting too many calories by the end of the week.

DAY 34

	Calories	Fat (g)	Carbs (g)	Protein (g)	Sugar (g)	Simple Sugar (g)
Breakfast						
3-egg omelet	220	15	1	20	0	
with ½ C. (80 g) diced tomato	16	0	3	1	2.5	
and ½ C. (80 g) spinach	37	2	4	3	0	
1 slice mozzarella cheese	86	5.5	1	7	0	
1 C. (150 g) assorted fruit	80	0	20	1	14	
12-oz. (350-ml) caffeinated or decaf coffee or tea, or water						
Breakfast totals	**439**	**22.5**	**29**	**32**	**16.5**	**0**
Midmorning Snack						
¼ C. (30 g) almonds	206	18	7	8	2	
1 medium banana	105	0	27	1	14	
8-oz. (240-ml) drink						
Snack totals	**311**	**18**	**34**	**9**	**16**	**0**
Lunch						
Turkey sandwich (4 slices)	120	2	4	20	4	
2 slices wholemeal bread	256	4	48	8	4	
2 slices tomato	7	0	2	0	1	
1 T. low-fat mayo	49	5	1	0	1	1
1 C. (150 g) raw veggies	25	0.25	6	1	3	
16-oz. (480-ml) decaf drink						
Lunch totals	**457**	**11.25**	**61**	**29**	**13**	**1**
Dinner						
8-oz. (230-g) tuna steak	180	2	0	40	0	
with 1 T. low-fat lemon dill sauce	130	6	6	1	2	2
6 spears asparagus	18	0	6	2	0	
1 T. extra-virgin olive oil	120	14	0	0	0	
2½ C. (100 g) romaine lettuce	15	0	3	1	1	
with 1½ T. balsamic vinaigrette	38	1.5	6	0	2	2
and 10 small black olives	36	3	2	0	0	
1 C. (120 g) sliced strawberries	53	0.5	13	1	8	

	Calories	Fat (g)	Carbs (g)	Protein (g)	Sugar (g)	Simple Sugar (g)
1 T. unsweetened Greek yogurt	25	1.5	2	0	1	1
16-oz. (480-ml) decaf drink						
Dinner totals	**615**	**33.5**	**38**	**45**	**18**	**5**
Evening Snack						
50-g protein shake	200	0	0	50	0	
½ medium banana	52	0	14	0.5	5	5
2 T. sugar-free chocolate syrup (8 oz./240 ml liquid total in shake)	15	0	5	1	0	
Snack totals	**267**	**0**	**19**	**51.5**	**7**	**5**
Day 34 totals	**2,089 cal**	**86 g**	**181 g**	**167 g**	**72 g**	**11 g**
		774 cal	724 cal	668 cal		
		37%	34%	31%		

DAY 35

	Calories	Fat (g)	Carbs (g)	Protein (g)	Sugar (g)	Simple Sugar (g)
Breakfast						
4-oz. (115-g) fillet steak	240	11	0	22	0	
2 scrambled eggs	144	10	1	12	0	
1 slice wholemeal toast	128	2	24	4	2	
5 oz. (145 g) unsweetened Greek yogurt	80	0	0	15	5	5
1 large orange	86	0	22	2	17	
12-oz. (350-ml) caffeinated or decaf coffee or tea, or water						
Breakfast totals	**678**	**23**	**47**	**55**	**24**	**5**
Midmorning Snack						
¼ C. (30 g) almonds	206	18	7	8	2	
12 oz. (350 ml) water						
Snack totals	**206**	**18**	**7**	**8**	**2**	**0**
Lunch						
4-oz. (115-g) veggie burger wrapped in lettuce	201	7	16	19	1	
with 1 t. ketchup	5	0	1	0	1	1

	Calories	Fat (g)	Carbs (g)	Protein (g)	Sugar (g)	Simple Sugar (g)
2 medium apples	144	0	38	0	28	
16-oz. (480-ml) decaf iced tea or water						
Lunch totals	**350**	**7**	**55**	**19**	**30**	**1**
Dinner						
Two 4-oz. (115-g) tilapia fillets	186	2	0	42	0	
2 C. (320 g) spinach, cooked	148	8	14	10	2	
1 medium baked potato with:	121	0	28	3	2	2
1 T. regular sour cream	27	3	0	0	0	
1 C. (100 g) grapes	110	0	29	1	25.	
16-oz. (480-ml) decaf iced tea or water						
Dinner totals	**592**	**13**	**71**	**56**	**29**	**2**
Evening Snack						
40-g pre-made protein shake (total 14 oz./400 ml liquid)	220	3	7	40	2	2
Snack totals	**220**	**3**	**7**	**40**	**2**	**2**
Day 35 totals	**2,046 cal**	**64 g**	**187 g**	**178 g**	**88 g**	**10 g**
		576 cal	748 cal	712 cal		
		28%	37%	35%		

Phase 3/Week 6 Shopping List

One dozen medium eggs

Wholemeal bread or
   wholemeal English muffins

Reduced sugar jam

Three medium oranges

Two 23-gram protein bars
   (such as Pure Protein
   brand)

Fresh watermelon

Ingredients for avocado
   tuna salad (recipe on
   page 262)

Four medium apples

16 ounces (450 grams)
   scallops

Sundried tomatoes

Extra-virgin olive oil

Brown rice

Fresh broccoli

Romaine lettuce

Black olives

Low-fat cottage cheese

Fresh strawberries,
   blueberries, raspberries,
   and other fresh fruit

Sugar-free ice cream

Three medium tomatoes

Natural peanut butter

Fresh spinach

Three 40-gram pre-made
   protein shakes (such as
   Muscle Milk)

6 ounces (170 grams) smoked
   salmon for salmon sushi
   (recipe on page 266)

Soy sauce

Romaine lettuce and rocket
   mix

Five cherry tomatoes

8-ounce (230-gram) tuna
   steak

8-ounce (230-gram) bottle
   of low-fat lemon dill sauce

Fresh asparagus spears

Unsweetened fat-free Greek
   yogurt

8-ounce (230-gram) bag
   almonds

Four medium bananas

Eight slices deli turkey breast

Low-fat mayonnaise

Assorted raw veggies
   (1 cup/150 grams)

5-ounce (145-gram) boneless
   pork chop

Two 6-ounce (170-gram)
   skinless chicken breasts

Red wine vinegar

Whole-wheat pasta

Whole-grain cereal

Rye bread

Dijon mustard

4-ounce (115-gram) fillet
   steak

Two medium baking potatoes

8-ounce (230-gram) tilapia
   fillet

Garlic salt

Cinnamon

One medium sweet potato

Butter

Protein powder (such as
   Isopure)

Skimmed or almond milk

Whole-grain pancake mix

Sugar-free maple syrup

Six slices lean deli roast beef

One tomato basil tortilla
   wrap

One slice cheddar cheese

Wholemeal pita crisps

Fresh grapes

8-ounce (230-gram) snapper
   fillet

Lemon pepper

Fresh mushrooms

Phase 3/Week 6 Daily Menus

DAY 36

	Calories	Fat (g)	Carbs (g)	Protein (g)	Sugar (g)	Simple Sugar (g)
Breakfast						
3 scrambled eggs	220	15	1	20	0	
1 slice wholemeal toast	128	2	24	4	2	
½ t. reduced sugar jam	8	0	3	0	2	2

	Calories	Fat (g)	Carbs (g)	Protein (g)	Sugar (g)	Simple Sugar (g)
1 large orange	85	0	21	1	17	
12-oz. (350-ml) caffeinated or decaf coffee or tea, or water						
Breakfast totals	**441**	**17**	**43**	**25**	**21**	**2**
Midmorning Snack						
23-g protein bar	200	6	16	23	3	3
12-oz. (350-ml) decaf drink						
Snack totals	**200**	**6**	**16**	**23**	**3**	**3**
Lunch						
1 C. (200 g) chicken/turkey/tuna salad (made with 1 T. low-fat mayo)	383	10	14.5	30	2	2
1 medium apple OR 2 C. (300 g) diced watermelon	80	0	21	1	14	
16-oz. (480-ml) decaf coffee, decaf tea, or water						
Lunch totals	**702**	**31**	**72**	**39**	**18**	**2**
Dinner						
8 oz. (230 g) baked scallops	300	7	6	42	0	
⅓ C. (20 g) sundried tomatoes	46	5	10	2.5	7	
1 T. extra-virgin olive oil	119	14	0	0	0	
½ C. (65 g) brown rice, cooked	108	2	22	3	1	
1 C. (225 g) broccoli	34	0	7	2	1	
2½ C. (100 g) romaine lettuce	15	0	3	1	1	
with 3 T. red wine vinegar	0	0	0	0	0	
and 5 small black olives	18	2	1	0	0	
½ C. (90 g) low-fat (1%) cottage cheese	81	1	3	14	3	3
with ½ C. (60 g) strawberries	27	0.25	7	0.5	4	
16-oz. (480-ml) decaf drink						
Dinner totals	**770**	**33**	**60**	**62**	**19**	**3**
Evening Snack						
2 t. sugar-free ice cream	50	1	5	0	0	
8-oz. (240-ml) sugar-free drink						
Snack totals	**50**	**1**	**5**	**0**	**0**	**0**

	Calories	Fat (g)	Carbs (g)	Protein (g)	Sugar (g)	Simple Sugar (g)
Day 36 totals	2,163 cal	86.5 g	198 g	149 g	61 g	10 g
		778.5 cal	792 cal	592 cal		
		36%	37%	27%		

DAY 37

	Calories	Fat (g)	Carbs (g)	Protein (g)	Sugar (g)	Simple Sugar (g)
Breakfast						
⅔ cup smoked salmon (90 g) with dash of lemon juice	106	4	0	16	0	
½ wholemeal bagel	150	1	26	5	1	
1 sliced medium apple	72	0	19	0	14	
1 T. peanut butter	100	8	3	4	1.5	1.5
8-oz. (240-ml) caffeinated or decaf coffee or tea, or water						
Breakfast totals	428	13	48	25	16.5	1.5
Midmorning Snack						
23-g protein bar	200	6	16	20	2	2
12-oz. (350-ml) decaf drink						
Snack totals	200	6	16	20	2	2
Lunch						
8-oz. (230-g) steak burger	560	45	0	40	0	
with 1 wholemeal bun	140	1	27	7	4	
and 1 T. ketchup	15	0	3.5	.25	3	3
4 sliced dill pickles	0	0	0	0	0	
½ cup (65 g) brown rice, cooked	108	0.5	22	5	0	
with 1 t. butter	33	3.5	0	0	0	
1 medium peach	38	0.25	9.5	1	8	
12-oz. (350-ml) decaf drink						
Lunch totals	894	51	61	54	15	3
Dinner						
2 small lamb chops, grilled and seasoned to taste	224	11	0	32	0	
½ T. barbecue sauce	35	0	9	0	8	8

	Calories	Fat (g)	Carbs (g)	Protein (g)	Sugar (g)	Simple Sugar (g)
1 C. (200 g) grilled veggies	25	0	4	2	1	
1 T. extra-virgin olive oil	120	14	0	0	0	
16-oz. (480-ml) decaf drink						
Dinner totals	**404**	**25**	**16**	**34**	**9**	**8**
Evening Snack						
½ C. (60 g) sliced strawberries	40	0	10	0	8	
with 1 T. unsweetened Greek yogurt	20	1	3	0	0	
mixed with 5 g protein powder	20	0	0	5	0	
12-oz. (350-ml) decaf drink						
Snack totals	**80**	**1**	**13**	**5**	**8**	**0**
Day 37 totals	**2,006 cal**	**96 g**	**151 g**	**134 g**	**50.5 g**	**14.5 g**
		864 cal	**604 cal**	**536 cal**		
		43%	**30%**	**27%**		

DAY 38

	Calories	Fat (g)	Carbs (g)	Protein (g)	Sugar (g)	Simple Sugar (g)
Breakfast						
3-egg omelet	220	15	1	20	0	
with ¼ C. (40 g) spinach and ¼ C. (40 g) diced tomato	20	1	3	3	2	
½ slice wholemeal toast	64	1	12	2	1	
1 T. peanut butter	100	8	3	4	1.5	1.5
1 large sliced orange	86	0	22	2	17	
12-oz. (350-ml) caffeinated or decaf coffee or tea, or water						
Breakfast totals	**490**	**25**	**39**	**31**	**21.5**	**1.5**
Midmorning Snack						
40-g pre-made protein shake	220	3	7	40	2	2
Snack totals	**220**	**3**	**7**	**40**	**2**	**2**

	Calories	Fat (g)	Carbs (g)	Protein (g)	Sugar (g)	Simple Sugar (g)
Lunch						
Salmon sushi made with 6 oz. (170 g) smoked salmon	396	15	0	63	0	
and ½ C. (65 g) brown rice, cooked	108	0.5	22	5	0	
2 C. (80 g) romaine lettuce and rocket mix	12	0	2	1	1	
with 5 cherry tomatoes	15	0	3	1	2	
and 5 small black olives	18	1.5	1	0	0	
2 T. soy sauce	20	0	0	2	1	1
12-oz. (350-ml) sugar-free drink						
Lunch totals	**569**	**17**	**28**	**72**	**4**	**1**
Dinner						
8-oz. (230-g) tuna steak	180	2	0	40	0	
with 2 T. low-fat lemon dill sauce	130	11	6	1	4	4
6 spears asparagus	18	0	6	2	0	
1 T. extra virgin olive oil	120	14	0	0	0	
1 C. (120 g) sliced strawberries	53	0.5	13	1	8	
1 T. unsweetened Greek yogurt	25	1.5	2	0	1	1
16-oz. (480-ml) sugar-free drink						
Dinner totals	**526**	**29**	**27**	**44**	**13**	**5**
Evening Snack						
¼ C. (30 g) almonds	206	18	7	8	2	
12-oz. (350-ml) decaf drink						
Snack totals	**206**	**18**	**7**	**8**	**2**	**0**
Day 38 totals	2,011 cal	92 g	108 g	195 g	42.5 g	9.5 g
		828 cal	432 cal	780 cal		
		41%	22%	38%		

DAY 39

	Calories	Fat (g)	Carbs (g)	Protein (g)	Sugar (g)	Simple Sugar (g)
Breakfast						
3-egg omelet	220	15	1	20	0	
with ½ C. (80 g) diced tomato	16	0	3	1	2.5	
and ½ C. (80 g) spinach	37	2	4	3	0	
1 slice mozzarella cheese	86	5.5	1	7	0	
1 C. (150 g) assorted fruit	80	0	20	1	14	
12-oz. (350-ml) caffeinated or decaf coffee or tea, or water						
Breakfast totals	**439**	**22.5**	**29**	**32**	**16.5**	**0**
Midmorning Snack						
¼ C. (30 g) almonds	206	18	7	8	2	
1 medium banana	105	0	27	1	14	
8-oz. (240-ml) drink						
Snack totals	**311**	**18**	**34**	**9**	**16**	**0**
Lunch						
Turkey sandwich (4 slices)	120	2	4	20	4	
2 slices wholemeal bread	256	4	48	8	4	
2 slices medium tomato	7	0	2	0	1	
1 T. low-fat mayo	49	5	1	0	1	1
1 C. (150 g) raw veggies	25	0.25	6	1	3	
16-oz. (480-ml) decaf drink						
Lunch totals	**457**	**11.25**	**61**	**29**	**13**	**1**
Dinner						
5-oz. (145-g) boneless pork chop	166	3	0	32	0	
with 1 T. low-fat lemon dill sauce	130	6	6	1	2	2
6 spears asparagus	18	0	6	2	0	
1 T. extra virgin olive oil	120	14	0	0	0	
2½ C. (100 g) romaine lettuce	15	0	3	1	1	
with 1½ T. balsamic vinaigrette	38	1.5	6	0	2	2
and 10 small black olives	36	3	2	0	0	
1 C. (120 g) sliced strawberries	53	0.5	13	1	8	

	Calories	Fat (g)	Carbs (g)	Protein (g)	Sugar (g)	Simple Sugar (g)
1 T. unsweetened Greek yogurt	25	1.5	2	0	1	1
16-oz. (480-ml) decaf drink						
Dinner totals	**601**	**34.5**	**38**	**37**	**18**	**5**
Evening Snack						
50-g protein shake	200	0	0	50	0	
½ small to medium banana	52	0	14	0.5	5	5
2 T. sugar-free chocolate syrup (8 oz./240 ml liquid total in shake)	15	0	5	1	0	
Snack totals	**267**	**0**	**19**	**51.5**	**7**	**5**
Day 39 totals	2,075 cal	87 g	181 g	159 g	72 g	11 g
		783 cal	724 cal	636 cal		
		38%	35%	31%		

DAY 40

	Calories	Fat (g)	Carbs (g)	Protein (g)	Sugar (g)	Simple Sugar (g)
Breakfast						
3-egg omelet	220	15	1	20	0	
with ¼ C. (40 g) spinach and ¼ C. (40 g) diced tomato	20	1	3	3	2	
½ slice wholemeal toast	64	1	12	2	1	
1 T. peanut butter	100	8	3	4	1.5	1.5
1 large sliced orange	86	0	22	2	17	
12-oz. (350-ml) caffeinated or decaf coffee or tea, or water						
Breakfast totals	**490**	**25**	**39**	**31**	**21.5**	**1.5**
Midmorning Snack						
40-g pre-made protein shake (14 oz./400 ml liquid total in shake)	220	3	7	40	2	2
Snack totals	**220**	**3**	**7**	**40**	**2**	**2**
Lunch						
Two 6-oz. (170-g) chicken breasts	405	18	0	72	0	
with 2½ C. (100 g) chopped romaine lettuce	15	0	3	1	1	

	Calories	Fat (g)	Carbs (g)	Protein (g)	Sugar (g)	Simple Sugar (g)
and 1½ T. extra-virgin olive oil	180	21	0	0	0	
and 3 T. red wine vinegar	0	0	0	0	0	
and 1 T. Parmesan cheese	22	1.5	0.2	2	0	
and 10 small black olives	36	3.25	2	0	0	
1 medium apple	72	0	19	0	14	
16-oz. (480-ml) decaf drink						
Lunch totals	**730**	**44**	**24.2**	**74**	**15**	**0**
Dinner						
8 oz. (230 g) baked scallops	300	7	6	42	0	
over 1 C. (115 g) whole-wheat pasta, cooked	174	1	37	7.5	1	
with 1 T. extra-virgin olive oil	120	14	0	0	0	
1 C. (225 g) steamed broccoli	34	0	7	2	1	
16-oz. (480-ml) decaf drink						
Dinner totals	**628**	**23**	**50**	**51.5**	**2**	**0**
Evening Snack						
1 C. (150 g) fresh fruit	46	0	11	1	9	
8-oz. (240-ml) decaf drink						
Snack totals	**46**	**0**	**11**	**1**	**9**	**0**
Day 40 totals	**2,114 cal**	**95 g**	**111 g**	**197.5 g**	**49.5 g**	**3.5 g**
		855 cal	444 cal	788 cal		
		40%	22%	37%		

DAY 41

	Calories	Fat (g)	Carbs (g)	Protein (g)	Sugar (g)	Simple Sugar (g)
Breakfast						
1 C. (30 g) whole-grain cereal	125	0	26	3	5	
¼ C. (60 ml) skimmed milk (always okay to swap almond milk with skimmed milk anywhere in the plan)	21	0	3	2	3	3
½ medium banana	50	0	13	1	7	
¼ C. (30 g) blueberries	41	0	10	0.5	7	

	Calories	Fat (g)	Carbs (g)	Protein (g)	Sugar (g)	Simple Sugar (g)
16-oz. (480-ml) caffeinated or decaf coffee or tea, or water						
Breakfast totals	**237**	**0**	**52**	**6.5**	**23**	**3**
Midmorning Snack						
4 slices turkey breast	90	2	4	15	3	
1 slice rye bread	83	1	15	3	1	1
with light glaze of Dijon mustard	2	0	0	0	0	
12-oz. (350-ml) sugar-free drink						
Snack totals	**175**	**3**	**19**	**18**	**4**	**1**
Lunch						
4-oz. (115-g) grilled fillet steak	240	11	0	22	0	
with 1 T. extra-virgin olive oil	120	14	0	0	0	
1 medium baked potato	120	0	28	3	1	1
½ C. (60 g) grilled asparagus	13	0	2	1.5	1	
12-oz. (350-ml) sugar-free drink						
Lunch totals	**493**	**25**	**30**	**26.5**	**2**	**1**
Dinner						
8-oz. (230-g) grilled tilapia fillet seasoned with garlic salt and cinnamon	220	4	0	45.5	0	
in 2 T. extra virgin olive oil	240	28	0	0	0	
2 C. (320 g) steamed spinach	14	0.25	2	2	0.25	
½ medium sweet potato	51	0	12	1.5	3	3
with 1 T. butter	100	11	1.5	0	1.5	1.5
½ C. (60 g) strawberries	26	0	7	0.5	4	
12-oz. (350-ml) decaf coffee, tea, or water						
Dinner totals	**650**	**39.25**	**22.5**	**49.5**	**8.75**	**4.5**
Evening Snack						
60-g protein shake	280	1	7	60	2	2
1 T. sugar-free caramel syrup	45	0	12	0	0	
¼ C. (60 ml) skimmed milk (always okay to swap almond milk with skimmed milk anywhere in the plan)	21	0	3	2	3	3

	Calories	Fat (g)	Carbs (g)	Protein (g)	Sugar (g)	Simple Sugar (g)
¼ C. (60 ml) almond milk	10	0	0.3	0.4	0	
1 C. (140 g) ice						
Snack totals	**356**	**1**	**22.3**	**62.4**	**5**	**5**
Day 41 totals	1,911 cal	71.25 g	146 g	153 g	44 g	14.5 g
		641 cal	584 cal	612 cal		
		34%	31%	32%		

DAY 42

	Calories	Fat (g)	Carbs (g)	Protein (g)	Sugar (g)	Simple Sugar (g)
Breakfast						
2 whole-grain pancakes	160	4	30	3.5	7	
mixed with 20 g protein powder	80	0	0	20	0	
with ½ C. (60 g) blueberries or ½ sliced small banana	83	0	21	1	14	
4 T. sugar-free maple syrup	10	0	4	0	0	
½ medium orange	31	0	7	1	6	
12-oz. (350-ml) caffeinated or decaf coffee or tea, or water						
Breakfast totals	**364**	**4**	**56**	**25.5**	**27**	**0**
Midmorning Snack						
¼ C. (30 g) almonds	206	18	7	8	2	
12-oz. (350-ml) sugar-free drink						
Snack totals	**206**	**18**	**7**	**8**	**2**	**0**
Lunch						
Roast beef wrap (6 slices)	336	20	0	33	0	
with tomato basil tortilla wrap	210	4.5	35	6	4	4
1 T. Dijon mustard	4	0	0.5	0.25	0	
1 slice cheddar cheese	70	6	0	4	0	
7 wholemeal pita crisps	110	3	18	4	0.5	0.5
½ C. (100 g) grapes	55	0	15	1	25	
12-oz. (350-ml) sugar-free drink						
Lunch totals	**795**	**24.5**	**68.5**	**48.25**	**29**	**4.5**

	Calories	Fat (g)	Carbs (g)	Protein (g)	Sugar (g)	Simple Sugar (g)
Dinner						
8-oz. (230-g) snapper fillet	227	3	0	46.5	0	
grilled with lemon pepper and 1 T. extra-virgin olive oil	120	14	0	0	0	
1 medium baked potato	121	0	28	3	2	2
1 t. butter	32	2.5	1	1.5	0.5	0.5
½ C. (90 g) mushrooms	7.5	0	1	1	0.5	
1 C. (160 g) spinach with garlic, cooked	74	4	7	5	1	
½ C. (60 g) blueberries/raspberries	83	0	21	1	14	
16-oz. (480-ml) decaf drink						
Dinner totals	**664.5**	**23.5**	**58**	**58**	**18**	**2.5**
Evening Snack						
40-g pre-made protein shake (14 oz./400 ml liquid total in shake)	220	3	7	40	2	2
Snack totals	**220**	**3**	**7**	**40**	**2**	**2**
Day 42 totals	**2,249.5 cal**	**72.5 g**	**196.5 g**	**180 g**	**78 g**	**8.5 g**
		652 cal	784 cal	720 cal		
		29%	35%	32%		

Chapter 6

The Exercise Bonanza

I begin this chapter by telling you about two very different people, Martina and Chelsea. Martina enjoyed indulging herself with a high-sugar diet, knowing she could burn off all the excess calories at the gym. Chelsea had never liked exercise, but for as long as she could remember she had eaten "low carb" *and* "low fat."

In other words, Martina wanted to manage her weight solely through exercise, while Chelsea wanted to manage her weight solely through diet. Let's see how each woman got along.

Martina's Story: Relying Solely on Exercise

A dynamic, energetic woman in her mid-forties, Martina had always been, in her own words, "a gym rat." Every morning before work, she ran ten miles (about 16 kilometres). Every evening after work, she put in two hours at the gym, doing high-level resistance training. Her vigorous workout schedule seemed to give her the leeway to indulge frequently in crisps, chips, and her favorite breakfast: a big bowl of porridge studded with raisins, swimming in warm full-fat milk, and covered with two spoonfuls of brown sugar.

Then Martina tore a ligament in her left knee, which required a complicated surgery and a three-month recovery. "Except for hobbling back and forth to work, I had nothing to do but eat," she told me ruefully. By the time Martina was back on her feet, she had gained fifteen pounds (almost 7 kilos).

Martina was sure that once she restarted her old exercise routine, the weight would come off easily. Instead, she found herself unable to lose much at all—and then, to her great concern, she began to gain even more.

Looking for diet advice in her favorite magazine, Martina read that she should cut back on both fats and carbs. Determined to get back to her healthy weight, Martina cut out the "high-carb" porridge, replacing it with a "low-carb" power bar, a skimmed latte, and a glass of freshly squeezed juice.

"And that's when my problems *really* started," Martina told me. Although her "low-carb," "low-fat," low-calorie breakfast was supposed to meet all her nutritional needs, Martina found herself ravenous by 10 o'clock in the morning. She tried to tough it out by having another skimmed latte, and when that didn't work, she had a second power bar. That kept her satisfied for about an hour—and then she was ravenous again. When she didn't eat, Martina told me, she felt dizzy and anxious, "like I really am starving."

When Martina finished her story, she looked at me anxiously. "I hate feeling so out of control," she said. "But I *really* want to lose weight. Do I just have to starve until I'm back in shape?"

Chelsea's Story: Relying Solely on Diet

Chelsea had never liked exercise. When she came to see me, she told me that she would follow any diet plan I offered, but she absolutely refused to consider any type of fitness program.

At the same time, Chelsea told me longingly about her best friend, Abby, whom she'd known since college.

"Abby has terrific genes," Chelsea said wistfully. "If I eat a brownie, it goes straight to my hips. But Abby has dessert at least once or twice a week, plus she has bread with her meals—bread! I can't even imagine doing that anymore. It must be nice to have genes like that . . ."

I asked Chelsea a little more about her lucky friend, and, as I suspected, Abby had always been physically active. In college, in fact, she had had a weight problem—she and Chelsea used to go on diets together. Then, during their junior year, Abby got interested in running. She started training for the long-distance running club at their college, and by their senior year, she was fit and at a healthy weight. Abby had taken up different types of exercise since then—problems with her knees had caused her to switch from long-distance running to brisk walking, occasional bike rides, and a regular resistance routine at the gym—but she had always remained physically active.

"Abby's terrific metabolism doesn't come from her genes," I told Chelsea. "You told me yourself that she was overweight in college. There are two reasons why Abby can indulge a bit more and still stay slim. First, from what you tell me, she never *over*indulges. She mainly eats a healthy diet and then every so often has a little something extra. Second, she stays active—not in an extreme way, but in a steady, moderate way. That helps to build muscle, and that muscle keeps her metabolism running in high gear."

Chelsea looked at me in surprise. She had never heard the problem broken down that way before.

"The great thing about this," I went on, "is that you can do exactly what Abby did, and you can get exactly the same results. Follow an eating plan that is high in protein and low in simple sugars, exercise moderately but steadily, and eventually, you'll have the metabolism of a teenager, just like your friend."

Chelsea shook her head. "But I hate exercise!"

I looked at her sympathetically. "I know you have never liked it. But when you follow my Appetite Solution, you won't be starting any exercise plan for the first two weeks. And I think when this new way of eating brings down your inflammation and you feel a lot more energetic, you'll feel ready to move."

The Problems with Too Much Exercise

From what you've read in this book so far, you probably already have a good idea of what's been going wrong for Martina:

- ☐ **Adaptive thermogenesis** and the *stress response* have caused her body to react with alarm to the unaccustomed exercise after her recovery. In response, her body is holding on to every bit of fat for dear life, and her appetite is going wild. True, Martina *used* to exercise at that intense level, but the three-month break caused her metabolism to reset.
- ☐ When Martina cuts back from a breakfast that is super-high in simple sugars (the raisins, sugar, and full-fat milk that she put on her porridge), her blood sugar levels drop—another reason she feels ravenous.
- ☐ Even though Martina's new breakfast is lower in simple sugars than her old one, it is still loaded with simple sugars (power bars, orange juice, skimmed milk), which are triggering an insulin response that cues her body to store fat—and that also keeps her perpetually hungry.

Like many people, Martina relied on exercise to make up for the unintended mistakes she made with her fork. For years, she ate a diet that was way too high in simple sugars and had more calories than she really needed. But by exercising to the extreme, she could hold off the effects of these dietary blunders.

Then an injury forced her to stop exercising. I've seen something similar with many of my patients, whether it's an injury, an illness, or the body wearing out from all that extreme exercise. Your body was simply not designed to be worked that hard, and sooner or later, you have to slow down. And the moment you do, your metabolism begins to stagger under the weight of all those extra calories and simple sugars.

To add insult to injury, the excessive rate at which Martina had been exercising was creating long-term stress for her body. Exercise in moderation is terrific for your health, but overdoing it is not. If your goal is to live a long, healthy, and vigorous life, looking terrific and feeling fabulous, too much exercise can be as bad as too little.

So for Martina, there was no going back to her old reliance on excessive exercise. She could no longer fix at the gym the choices she made with her fork. She was going to have to find a new way to move forward.

And so she did. At my advice, she began a moderate but still vigorous exercise plan—one that pushed her body but did not overstress it. She also followed the three phases of the Appetite Solution, boosting protein quickly and cutting simple sugars gradually, and, finally, rebalancing her metabolism and transforming her appetite.

To her delight, the extra weight came off smoothly and easily, her appetite became mild and pleasant, and the new fitness plan left her feeling energized, calm, and satisfied. "I think I'm actually in better shape now than when I was pushing myself so hard," she told me during her last visit. "It feels great to finally feel healthy!"

The Problem with Too Little Exercise

Chelsea was facing a different challenge. We have already seen why a restrictive diet makes it almost impossible to lose weight, so Chelsea's first step was to switch from her lifetime of restrictive diets to the more effective approach of the Appetite Solution. After years of avoiding carbs like the plague, it took Chelsea a little while to get used to the idea that I actually *wanted* her to eat wholemeal toast and brown rice, but once she understood the biology, she was ready to get on board.

What was harder for Chelsea was accepting that exercise had to be part of the solution.

"Why can't I just eat less?" she kept asking me. "Then I wouldn't have to exercise."

Now let me be clear about this: If your only goal is to lose a few pounds, you don't *have* to exercise. If you follow the Appetite Solution, you *can* lose weight through diet alone, first loading up on protein, then cutting the simple sugars, all without a severe drop in calories.

However, to *keep* weight off easily—let alone to achieve the metabolism of a teenager—exercise is crucial. Not the extreme exercise that Martina favored, but moderate exercise, at least four times a week, for about thirty minutes each session. That will be your best weight-prevention tool going forward.

Why?

☐ **Exercise builds lean muscle mass.** As we have seen, lean muscle burns more calories. The lower your proportion of body fat and the higher your proportion of muscle, the more calories you burn— even while you are sleeping or watching TV.

☐ **Exercise reduces inflammation.** Inflammation cues your body to store fat. Reducing inflammation cues your body to burn fat. Anything you can do to reduce inflammation is enormously helpful for weight loss. And exercise—in moderation—is one of the best, most reliable ways to reduce inflammation that we know. (Ironically, Martina's extreme exercise was actually producing inflammation.[32])

☐ **Exercise reduces stress.** Stress also cues your body to store fat. And exercise—again in moderation—is one of the best known ways to reduce stress. (Again, Martina's extreme exercise actually created stress.[33])

So, I told Chelsea, if she wanted to relax into her new healthy weight instead of having to remain super-vigilant with her diet, exercise was key. The danger she faced if she did *not* exercise was that some other source of stress or inflammation—a massive deadline at work, a fight with her boyfriend, a bout with the flu, or even a momentary slip in her dietary discipline—would set her up for weight gain once again.

The real challenge for Chelsea was how much she hated even the thought of exercise. I asked her to hang in there and give it time. For the first two weeks of the Appetite Solution, I told her, she would focus on the food and ignore exercise altogether. I didn't want to trigger adaptive thermogenesis or the stress response by having her do too much, too soon.

Two weeks in, I shared a moderate exercise program with Chelsea, one that was appropriate for someone who was not used to exercising and who felt daunted by the very idea. Because she had been following the Appetite Solution for two weeks, Chelsea did feel more energized than she had felt in a long time, so she agreed to give my exercise program a try.

To her surprise, Chelsea actually liked the way exercise made her feel. She noticed that her mood was better and that she felt "less stressed." She also noticed that her clothes fit differently because her body was "tighter," as she put it. All of that gave her motivation to continue.

Chelsea lost the weight she wanted to and continued with both the eating plan and the fitness plan that I recommended. I stopped seeing her when she reached her healthy weight, but several months later, she called me in delight.

"I never really believed I could get the metabolism of a teenager," she told me, "but you were right, Dr. Colella, that's exactly what I have! Just like Abby, I can have dessert every so often, or some chips, or whatever, and I just burn it off right away. As long as I stick to the plans you gave me, I know I'll stay at this weight. What a relief!"

Your Appetite Solution Fitness Plans: Two Choices

Clearly, not everybody has the same relationship with exercise—and that's just fine. Whether you're a lifelong exerciser like Martina or a newcomer to the party like Chelsea, you can still achieve terrific results while you are following the Appetite Solution.

I've made things easier by developing two separate fitness plans, which you can find in chapter 7. If, like Chelsea, you are new to the idea of exercise, or if you believe you lack the physical fitness or mobility to do most workouts, follow the Chelsea Plan. If you like exercise, go to the gym even as often as a few times a month, or are doing some other form of semi-regular workout, follow the Martina Plan.

Both plans include a mix of cardiovascular and resistance training. Both plans enable you to burn significant amounts of calories—*and* to boost your metabolism by building more lean muscle mass. Meanwhile, the protein you'll consume as you follow the Appetite Solution will help your muscles grow even faster.

The combination of all those physiological responses put together is unbeatable. It leads not only to accelerated weight loss, but also prevents future weight gain. It's a win-win-win-win situation.

Cardio and Resistance Training

☐ **Cardiovascular exercise ("cardio")** includes brisk walking, running, elliptical training, cycling, swimming, or any type of activity that gets your heart pumping above its normal rate. Because your heart beats faster and your lungs need to breathe more deeply, cardio boosts your metabolism and is also terrific for your heart and lungs.

☐ **Resistance exercise** has you working against the resistance of either your own body's weight or other weight to develop your strength. As you work to increase your strength, you are also building lean muscle mass, which, as we have seen, gets your metabolism to burn more calories even when you are sleeping or at rest.

How Cardio Training Helps You Lose Weight

Cardio training gets its name from its effects on your heart, getting it to pump at a higher than normal rate. But a faster heart rate means that you are also working your lungs—forcing your body to do an activity just slightly past its ability to breathe normally. In technical terms, this is known as the *anaerobic* realm—the place where you are not getting quite enough oxygen.

Your body obviously depends upon air to live, however. So when you force it past the point of easy breathing, you spur a hormonal shift that, when you do it long enough and consistently enough—say, half an hour a day, three times a week, as when you are following the Appetite Solution fitness plan—you actually shift your metabolism. Your body begins to burn fat for energy, and the weight comes off more easily.

To some extent, cardio also builds muscle. Whether you're walking, swimming, using a treadmill, riding a stationary bike, or doing some other form of brisk, regular movement, you are also working your muscles, though not quite to the same extent as when you're doing resistance training. Nevertheless, the muscle you build through cardio also gets your metabolism humming, burning calories even while you are sleeping.

How Resistance Training Helps You Lose Weight

Here's the truly remarkable thing about resistance training: It keeps burning calories for up to thirty-six hours after you have stopped moving. In the early postexercise stages, you also consume extra oxygen in an attempt to bring your body temperature, heart rate, and blood oxygen levels back to normal.[34] Basically, you're breaking your muscles down and then building them back up again, and that process pushes your metabolism in an amazing way. I'm very excited for you to give your weight-loss efforts an enormous boost by adding resistance training to the mix.

The goal of resistance training is to use the big muscle groups of the body as frequently as possible to allow for both maximal calorie burn and maximal muscle growth. In my fitness plans, we'll be focusing on two teams of big muscles:

☐ Your thighs and glutes (the muscles in your butt)
☐ Your chest and shoulders

All of these muscles are anchored by your core, the muscles that wrap around the central part of your skeleton like a tightly wound rubber band. You always want to strengthen your core, because that's the basis of your whole body's strength. Working the two big-muscle groups that I am targeting will also help you achieve amazing core strength that will only get better over time.

Two key exercises work the two big muscle groups—and they don't even require any equipment! Whether you're following the Chelsea Plan or the Martina Plan, these two exercises will be your starting point for resistance training: the push-up and the squat. The push-ups work your upper body—your chest and shoulders—while the squats work your lower body—your thighs and glutes. I've designed the Appetite Solution fitness plans to work all of your big-muscle groups in a consistent manner.

Now, before you start to panic, there are many variations for each exercise, so they can be easily adapted to any fitness level. If you've never exercised in your life, you can start with a very simple wall push-up. If you've been exercising for years and think push-ups are too easy for you, I present some variations that will be more challenging. The same goes for squats. I've organized both exercise plans in such a way that you can easily find the right level for you—and then gradually work your way up to an even higher level of fitness.

Reps, Sets, and Circuits

For those of you who are new to the exercise game, the terminology can be unfamiliar. Here is everything you need to know.

The basic unit of a routine is called the *rep*, which is short for *repetition*. If I say, "do ten reps of wall push-ups," that means you repeat a wall push-up until you have done ten of them. Very rarely do you ever do just one of anything. Usually you do a few reps of a particular exercise. Repeating the exercise helps break down the muscle. Then your body uses protein to build it back up and make it even stronger. That process of breaking down and building up is where you get your metabolic benefits—and it all starts with the first rep.

The next unit is the *set*, which is a group of reps. For example, if you do ten wall push-ups (ten reps), that would be one set.

Finally, there is the *circuit*, which is a combination of sets. For example, if you do one set of push-ups (ten push-ups) followed by one set of squats (ten squats), that combination of push-ups and squats would be one circuit.

Your resistance workout will never last longer than thirty minutes, plus another few minutes for a warm-up. Your goal is to complete as much of the prescribed workout as possible within that thirty minutes. Each thirty-minute workout will burn a lot of calories—*and* it will keep burning them for the next one or two days.

Moving quickly from one set to the next, with no more than fifteen seconds of rest in between, will keep your heart rate up and your metabolism high. It basically means that you get both cardio *and* resistance benefits from your resistance training.

At this point, you might be wondering why you can't do *only* resistance training. The answer is simple: the stress response. You need to stress your muscles a little, to get them to grow, but you can't stress them too much, or you'll end up disrupting your metabolism in other ways. Also, since resistance training breaks your muscles down, you have to give your body time to repair them.

So here's your takeaway, and it applies whether you're a "Chelsea" or a "Martina," a novice or a gym rat:

☐ Too little resistance training deprives you of some terrific weight-loss benefits.

☐ Too much resistance training can overstress your body and make weight loss even more difficult.

☐ Your goal is to find the right amount of resistance training for your body as it is now—and then gradually increase your training as your body gets stronger.

More Reps Versus More Weight—Don't Get Hurt

A lot of people set their sights on lifting heavier and heavier weights. If your goal is to become the next body-building champion, that might be a good idea. But if your goal is to lose weight, you'll do way better with *less weight and more reps.* In other words, use a lighter weight but do more reps with it.

Many fitness experts believe that the combination of less weight and more reps burns more calories with less risk for injury than routines that use heavier weights. Adding reps might take a bit more time, but it is far more effective for creating the lean muscle mass your body needs to become a fat-burning machine. As an added benefit, less weight is way better for your joints and reduces the risk of an injury that could keep you from exercising altogether.

If you are already lifting weights, and you are still trying to lose weight, you are almost certainly using too much weight and not doing enough reps. When you begin your Appetite Solution fitness plan, a good rule of thumb is to drop your weight load by at least 30 percent and increase your number of reps by the same amount.

Let's suppose that you have been lifting 30-pound (13.6-kilo) dumb-bells in each hand for most of your arm exercises, and doing two sets of twelve reps. You would decrease those weights by 30 percent (9 pounds, or about 4 kilos) and begin lifting the closest barbell to that figure, which would be a 20-pound (9-kilo) weight. At the same time, you would increase your reps by 30 percent, which would increase your overall total reps by seven (30 percent of twenty-four). You would still do two sets, but of fifteen reps instead of twelve. Yes, you're lifting less weight—but you're burning more calories. And isn't that your goal?

Stick to Your Eating Plan

I've been telling you that exercise burns calories and boosts metabolism—and it does. But it will not accomplish those goals for you if you're loading up your diet with simple sugars or not eating enough protein. Please don't use your fitness plan as a reason to "cheat," indulge, swap foods, or deviate from your eating plan in any other way. The two plans work *together,* not separately. I'd hate for you to put in your time and energy with a fitness plan that you yourself were sabotaging with your fork.

Exercise: A Weight-Loss Triumph

As you increase the speed at which your body processes calories, you'll basically burn more calories as fuel and store fewer of them as fat. Hey, you just foiled adaptive thermogenesis! Not to mention reducing stress, boosting your mood, tightening up your body, and creating a whole bunch of other health benefits. If you want to lose weight, look terrific, and feel fabulous, exercise can be your new best friend. So turn the page and head on to chapter 7, where your Appetite Solution fitness plan awaits.

Your Appetite Solution
Fitness Plans

In this chapter, you'll find two Appetite Solution fitness plans. If you're new to exercise, haven't exercised in years, or are struggling with physical limitations, start with the kinder, gentler Chelsea Plan, starting on page 191. You'll get a terrific workout but one that will allow you to ease in to exercise gradually and improve at your own pace.

If you're used to exercise and looking for a more challenging workout, go to the more vigorous Martina Plan, beginning on page 198. You'll get a workout that allows you to increase your progress and that is specially geared toward helping you lose weight.

Before you start, however, I'd like to remind both groups of some basic fitness principles.

WARNING: Check with Your Doctor

Please consult with your doctor before beginning any new exercise plan to make sure that you are medically cleared for the amount of exertion that you hope to achieve.

Start Slow

The single most important guideline when it comes to any form of exercise is to avoid injury. This is a crucial basic priority that even experienced exercisers overlook, so let's take a few minutes for it here.

The two most common reasons why people stop following an exercise regimen are burnout and injury. I often see beginners trying to make up for years of inactivity in one super-vigorous workout—and then what happens? At worst, they're laid up with an injury that keeps them from exercising for still more days, weeks, or months. At best, they end up exhausted, setting off a stress reaction that triggers adaptive thermogenesis. Either way, their overexertion had the exact opposite of the effect they hoped to achieve.

Learn from their mistakes and start slow! Whether you're a first-time exerciser or a committed gym rat, doing too much, too soon can get you into trouble. Push yourself a little—but never too much.

Keep It Brisk

When you begin your resistance training, you want to perform each set at a fairly brisk pace, with no more than fifteen seconds of rest between sets. If you rest too long between sets, your heart rate returns to normal and you lose some of the extra calorie-burning benefits.

If you are a beginner, what does this mean for you? It means that always, my goal for you is to maintain moderate intensity rather than duration—that you should choose doing something briskly for a short time rather than with lots of pauses for a long time. I'd rather you stop after five minutes of brisk exercise than keep pausing and dragging yourself through the next exercise just to fill up the half hour.

I've given you thirty minutes for each resistance workout, but if you can't make it through the whole thirty minutes, stop when you feel that you should. Then the next time, stick it out a little longer . . . then a little longer . . . and eventually, you'll fill up the entire half hour with brisk, effective exercise. It doesn't matter how long it takes you to get there; the important thing is to keep moving and to keep improving, little by little. You'll get there in the end, and meanwhile, you're burning lots of calories on the journey!

Always Warm Up for Resistance Training

On resistance days it is crucial to always begin with a warm-up: at least five minutes of light cardio. A brisk walk will do it. At the gym, you can spend five minutes on the treadmill, the elliptical trainer, or a stationary bike. At home, if it's not practical to take a walk, march in place, bringing your knees up as high as you can and swinging your arms across your chest—crossing and then opening your arms. That's terrific low-impact cardio that you can do in place, and it makes a great warm-up.

Never neglect your warm-up. If necessary, take five minutes off your routine so that you have time to warm up. You need to get your joints lubricated and to increase the blood flow to your muscles before working out, or you could seriously injure yourself.

Your Workout Schedule

The most exercise you'll ever do for the Appetite Solution is half an hour a day, with a few more minutes to warm up for your resistance training. Ideally, you'll do five days of consecutive training and then rest for two days—that's the best schedule for weight loss. However, if you can't make five days in a row, do your best to reach any combination of five out of seven days. Alternate between cardio and resistance, with two days of cardio and three of resistance, every week. Here's a sample schedule:

Sample Workout Plan						
Monday	Tuesday	Wednesday	Thursday	Friday	Saturday	Sunday
Resistance circuits	Cardio	Resistance circuits	Cardio	Resistance circuits	Rest	Rest

However, to avoid confusion and keep yourself on track, pick a "first day of the week" that is always the same, and then reset the clock on that day. Let's say last week, you were down with the flu and couldn't exercise Monday, Tuesday, or Wednesday. You managed to get some training in on Thursday and Friday, but the weekend was packed with family obligations.

No worries. Take a deep breath and start again on Monday. Don't try to make up for missed workouts, and don't let a few missed workouts make you lose hope and give up entirely. Also, please don't say, "Oh, I've already missed my chance to have five workouts this week—I'll just wait till Monday and start over." Any workout is better than no workout.

Finally, if you have to do less than five workouts during any one week, focus on the resistance. If you can do only three workouts, for example, they should all be resistance workouts. That's where the weight-loss benefits truly are. Don't do any *more* than three resistance workouts—but try your best not to do any *less.*

Remember, your goal is to burn fat to achieve your ideal weight, while working your way toward the metabolism of a teenager. The combination of your diet plan and your fitness plan is how you'll get there . . . so keep your eyes on the prize!

A Schedule for Success

- ☐ Always warm up—even if you have to take time off your thirty minutes of training to do so.
- ☐ If you have to miss a workout, skip the cardio so you can do the resistance training.
- ☐ If you miss some time, just keep going . . . any workout is better than no workout.
- ☐ Reset the clock on your start day.

Should You Eat Before Your Workout?

There have been a lot of contradictory answers to this question, whether you look at the scientific research, the advice of professional trainers, or the personal experience of active people. After surveying the patients in my practice, as well as myself and my superathletic teenage sons, I've decided that the answer to this questions is very individual. You need to decide what works best for your body and stick to that.

So if you find that eating breakfast makes your workout feel easier, then eat something before beginning your routine. If you feel more powerful just on coffee or water alone, then stick to that.

I personally like to drink a protein shake either an hour or two before my workout or immediately after. However, if you feel weak during a workout, or if your stamina seems to be slipping, try a protein drink right then and there.

Exercise Descriptions

The following exercises are the building blocks for your fitness routine. Whether you're starting the Chelsea Plan or the Martina Plan, you can refer to these descriptions as you work your way through your plan.

Exercises You Can Do at Home

STANDARD BODY SQUAT

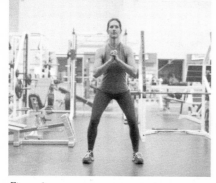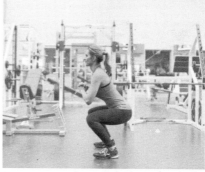

Figure 1

Stand up with good posture, with your feet slightly wider than shoulder width and your toes pointed forward. Clench your hands and hold them at your chest. Begin by bending your knees and sticking out your buttocks, lowering your trunk and upper body until your thighs are parallel with the floor at a roughly 90-degree angle. Keep your back as straight as possible. If necessary, place a chair behind you so that you are almost sitting down on it, which will also help you keep from falling.

LATERAL BODY SQUAT

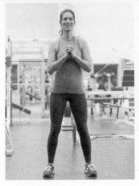
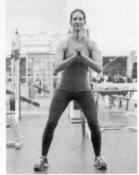
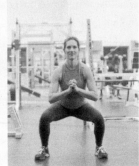

Figure 2

Start from the same position as the standard squat, this time extending one foot about 12 inches (30 centimetres) to either the right or left as you perform the squat and keeping your back as straight as possible. Alternate between left and right each time you do a squat. Once again, if you are a beginner, feel free to place a chair behind you.

STANDARD PUSH-UP

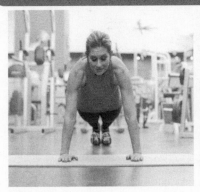
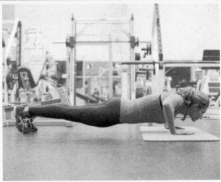

Figure 3

Lie facedown on the floor. Place your feet together and push your body up so that only your toes and your hands are touching the floor. Your body should be in a straight line with your knees stiff and your hands at shoulder width. Lower yourself slowly toward the floor until your chest is close to the floor. Then push back up to the starting position.

KNEE PUSH-UP

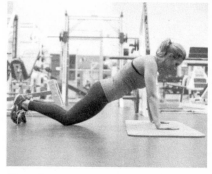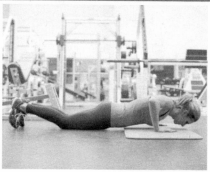

Figure 4

This push-up is slightly easier. Try if the standard push-up is too challenging when you begin. Kneel on the floor with your arms supporting your upper body, placed on the floor at shoulder width. Lower yourself slowly toward the floor until your chest is close to the floor. Then push back up to the starting position.

WALL PUSH-UP

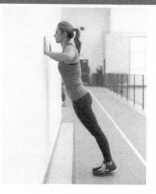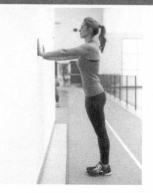

Figure 5

If the knee push-up doesn't work for you, the wall push-up certainly will. Stand at arm's length from the wall, feet together, back straight. Place your hands on the wall, shoulder width apart. As if doing a push-up, lean your body toward the wall, keeping your back straight as you bend your arms. Slowly straighten your arms to push yourself back into an upright position.

WIDE-HAND PUSH-UP

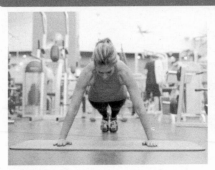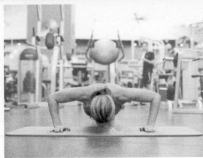

Figure 6

Starting from the standard push-up position, slowly work each hand out about 6 inches (15 centimetres) from your shoulders. Push yourself up, then lower yourself slowly until your chest is close to the floor.

CLOSE-HAND PUSH-UP

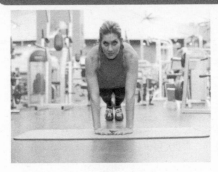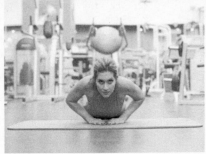

Figure 7

Starting from the standard push-up position, move each hand inward about 6 inches (15 centimetres). Push yourself up, then lower yourself slowly until your chest is close to the floor.

Exercises to Do at the Gym

Shoulder Stabilization

The following exercises will all help you stabilize your shoulders, thereby enhancing your ability to safely perform the other upper-body exercises in your plan. Maintain good form by keeping your wrist in the thumbs-up orientation (see photos for Cable Internal Rotation and Cable External Rotation). This will prevent rotator cuff impingement and keep your shoulders healthy and strong for whatever challenge is ahead.

CABLE INTERNAL ROTATION

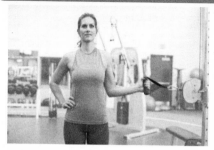 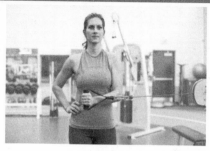

Figure 8

Stand facing a cable machine, at arm's length, your feet shoulder width apart. Hold the handle attached to the cable at a 90-degree angle from your body with your upper arm pressed against your body. Keep your forearm parallel to the floor and pull the handle to your body just below your breast bone. Hold for one second, then return to the starting position.

This exercise can also be performed with a resistance band.

CABLE EXTERNAL ROTATION

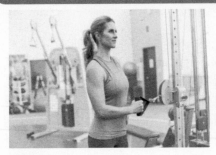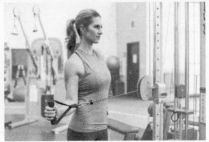

Figure 9

Stand with your back to a cable machine, at arm's length, your feet shoulder width apart. Hold the handle attached to the cable with the handle just below your breast bone, your arm bent at a 90-degree angle to your torso and the upper part of the arm pressed against your body. With your forearm parallel to the floor, pull the handle away from your body until the handle is in front of you, in line with your shoulder. Return to the starting position after holding for one second.

This exercise can also be performed with a resistance band.

INCLINE BENCH REVERSE FLY

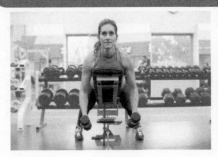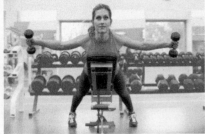

Figure 10

Lie facedown on an incline bench at a 30-degree angle with your face and neck extending above the top of the bench. Hold dumbbells in front of you under the bench, palms facing each other. With your elbows slightly bent, raise the dumbbells to the side until they are at shoulder height. Hold for one second and then return to the starting position.

UPRIGHT FORWARD SHOULDER EXTENSION

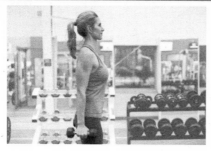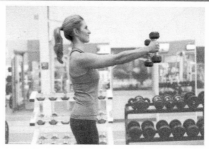

Figure 11

Stand upright, feet slightly more than shoulder width apart. Hold a dumbbell at your side with your palm facing your hip. With your elbow straight, raise the weight directly in front of you until it reaches shoulder height, keeping your palm and wrist position the same. Hold for one second and return to the starting position.

BENCH PRESS

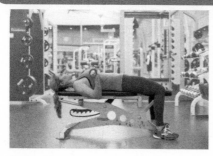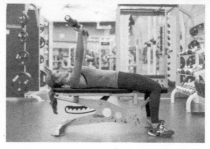

Figure 12

With a spotter: Lie on a flat bench holding a barbell with your hands slightly more than shoulder width apart, just above your nipple line. Slowly lower the bar until it is close to your chest. Hold for one second and then push the bar back to the starting position.

Or, solo: Use one of the fitness machine bench press equivalents at your gym.

INCLINE BENCH CRUNCH

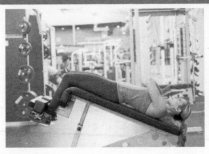 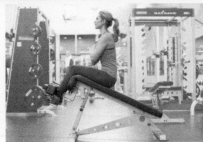

Figure 13

This is an advanced exercise, so if you have even the least doubt about how to do it, consult with an appropriately certified person at your gym. With a bench at a 30-degree incline and fitted with the appropriate pads to lock your feet and shins in place, lie on the bench facing the ceiling with your head at the low end of the bench and your legs, bent at the knees, draped over the top of the bench. Cross your arms over your chest and raise your chest until your upper body is perpendicular to the floor, hold for one second, and then return slowly to the starting position.

Alternatively, you can perform the same crunch lying flat on the floor with your knees bent at 90 degrees and raising your upper body off the floor, keeping your back flat and your chin off your chest.

STANDING BICEPS CURL

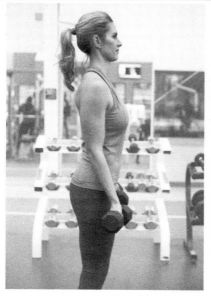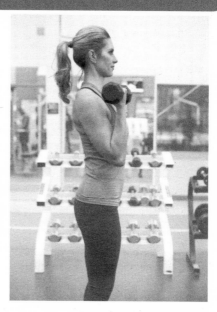

Figure 14

Stand upright, feet slightly more than shoulder width apart. Hold a dumbbell at your side with your palms facing forward. Keeping your upper arm close to your body, tuck your elbows into your side and raise the weight upward toward your shoulder. Hold for one second, then return to the starting position.

The Chelsea Plan

CHELSEA'S PHASE 1: WEEKS 1 AND 2

No Exercise

If you remember what I've said throughout this book about adaptive thermogenesis, you'll know why I'm having you hold off on the exercise for the first two weeks of the Appetite Solution.

First, I know it's hard to make too many changes at the same time. If you've never exercised much, I don't want you to have to focus on both diet and exercise. And I definitely don't want to trigger adaptive thermogenesis. If you feel like taking a brisk walk every now and then, go for it. Other than that, just focus on enjoying the high-protein meals of Phase 1.

CHELSEA'S PHASE 2: WEEKS 3 AND 4

CARDIO: twice a week

Week 3: Walk a quarter mile (0.4 kilometres) or twenty minutes, whichever takes you less time. Walk at a comfortable pace—don't push yourself. Your goal is to keep moving continuously, with no pauses to rest. If you have to slow down to accomplish that goal, slow down.

If you live in a city, a quarter mile (0.4 kilometres) is about five blocks. You can also measure the distance on the odometer of your car or use a smartphone app to measure the distance the first time you walk a new route.

Week 4: Walk half a mile (0.8 kilometres) or thirty minutes, whichever takes less time. Again, your goal is to keep moving, at whatever pace is right for you.

Of course, if you feel exhausted after even a few minutes of slow walking, please stop, get some rest, drink some water, and call it quits for the day. I don't want you exhausting yourself—that's only going to set up a stress response that keeps you from losing weight.

The important thing is to keep at it. Each day, walk a little more . . . then a little more . . . then a little more. Eventually, you will find yourself walking farther and faster, even if it takes you several weeks to get to that point. The rest of your Appetite Solution fitness plan follows here, but if you need to stretch out this beginning time for several weeks, listen to your body and don't stress.

RESISTANCE: three times a week

Week 3: Do as much of the following routine as you can comfortably complete in thirty minutes: three circuits.

One circuit: Ten standard push-ups followed immediately by ten squats. (Feel free to substitute knee or wall push-ups if you prefer.)

I don't want you resting more than about twenty seconds between circuits, and I don't want you overdoing it. So if you can't finish the whole thirty minutes without taking lots of long pauses—or if you can't finish more than a few push-ups in your first circuit—don't worry. Stop for the day, drink some water, and take it easy. Pick it up again the next resistance day, and keep trying. Little by little, you will improve.

Week 4: Do as much of the following routine as you can comfortably complete in thirty minutes: six circuits.

One circuit: Ten standard push-ups followed immediately by ten squats. (Feel free to substitute knee or wall push-ups if you prefer.)

Again, I don't want you resting more than about twenty seconds between circuits, and I don't want you overdoing it. Stop when you need to, and pick it up again the next time.

CHELSEA'S PHASE 3: WEEKS 5 AND 6

CARDIO: twice a week

Week 5: Walk 1 mile (1.6 kilometres) or thirty minutes, whichever takes less time.

Week 6: Walk 1½ miles (2.4 kilometres) or thirty minutes, whichever takes less time.

RESISTANCE: three times a week

Weeks 5 and 6: Do as much of the following routine as you can comfortably complete in thirty minutes: ten circuits.

One circuit: Ten standard push-ups followed immediately by ten squats. (Feel free to substitute knee or wall push-ups if you prefer.)

CHELSEA, BEYOND PHASE 3: WEEKS 7 AND 8

CARDIO: twice a week

Walk briskly or lightly jog, aiming for 2 miles (3.2 kilometres) in thirty minutes. It might take you a while to work your way up to this, but do your best here, and soon enough, your body will be wanting more!

If you have any arthritis or pain in your knees, hips, or ankles, DO NOT JOG: stick to walking.

RESISTANCE: three times a week

At this point, you'll want to work out at a gym for additional resistance benefits. The following workout focuses on shoulder stabilization and relies on weights and machines that you can find at any gym or fitness center.

- ☐ **Cable Internal Rotations:** Fifteen reps with very light weight (no more than 5 to 10 pounds/2.25 to 4.5 kilos)
- ☐ **Cable External Rotation:** Fifteen reps with very light weight (no more than 5 to 10 pounds/2.25 to 4.5 kilos)
- ☐ **Incline Bench Reverse Fly:** Two sets of twelve reps each; beginners should feel free to use 5-pound (2.25-kilo) dumbbells to start and increase the weight as you can. Rest for twenty seconds between sets.
- ☐ **Upright Forward Shoulder Extension:** Using 10- to 15-pound (4.5- to 6.8-kilo) dumbbells in each hand, do two sets of fifteen reps with twenty seconds of rest between sets.
- ☐ **Bench Press:** Three sets of eighteen to twenty reps with a weight that is one-third of your body weight. Rest only twenty seconds between sets.
- ☐ **Goblet Squat:** Three sets of eighteen to twenty reps with a weight that is one-quarter to one-fifth of your body weight. Rest only twenty seconds between sets.

   This exercise is performed exactly like a standard body squat except that you hold a dumbbell or kettlebell with both hands just in front of your chest below your chin.

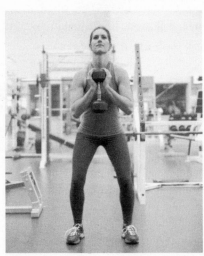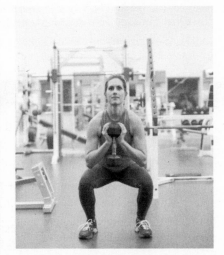

Figure 15

- ☐ **Incline Bench Crunch:** Set the bench at a 60-degree incline and do four sets of eighteen to twenty reps each. Be sure to cross your right shoulder to your left knee and vice versa for the last six reps of each set.

☐ **Standing Biceps Curl:** Four sets of eighteen to twenty reps with a weight that is no more than one-seventh of your body weight. Rest only twenty seconds between sets.

CHELSEA, BEYOND PHASE 3: LIFETIME

CARDIO: twice a week

Walk briskly or lightly jog, aiming for 2 miles (3.2 kilometres) in thirty minutes. At this point, feel free to mix in some new forms of cardio. For example: ten minutes of light jogging immediately followed by ten minutes on the elliptical, immediately followed by ten minutes of jumping rope.

Also feel free to do thirty minutes of swimming, stationary biking, or rowing.

RESISTANCE: three times a week

Alternate the upper-body workout with the lower-body workout, both described below. That is, one week, do two upper-body workouts and one lower-body workout, and the next week, do one upper-body workout and two lower-body workouts.

Upper-Body Workout

INCLINE BENCH CRUNCH

☐ Three sets of twenty reps. Vary the upper-body twist at the top of the crunch.

This is an advanced exercise, so if you have any doubt about how to do it, consult with an appropriately certified person at your gym.

With a bench at a 30-degree incline and fitted with the appropriate pads to lock your feet and shins in place, lie on the bench facing the ceiling with your head at the low end of the bench and your legs, bent at the knees, draped over the top of the bench. Cross your arms over your chest and raise your chest until your upper body is perpendicular to the floor, hold for one second, and then return slowly to the starting position.

Alternatively, you can perform the same crunch lying flat on the floor with your knees bent at 90 degrees and raising your upper body off the floor, keeping your back flat and your chin off your chest.

SHOULDER STABILIZATION

- ☐ **Cable Internal Rotations:** Fifteen reps with very light weight (no more than 5 to 10 pounds/2.25 to 4.5 kilos).
- ☐ **Cable External Rotation:** Fifteen reps with very light weight (no more than 5 to 10 pounds/2.25 to 4.5 kilos).
- ☐ **Incline Bench Reverse Fly:** Two sets of twelve reps each, using a weight that is comfortable from the previous phase; rest for twenty seconds between sets.
- ☐ **Upright forward shoulder extension:** Using 10- to 15-pound (4.5- to 6.8-kilo) dumbbells in each hand, do two sets of fifteen reps with twenty seconds of rest between sets.
- ☐ **Bench Press:** Four sets of eighteen to twenty reps with a weight that is one-third of your body weight. Rest only twenty seconds between sets.

PUSH-UPS

- ☐ Two sets of ten reps of standard push-ups
- ☐ Two sets of ten reps of wide-hand push-ups
- ☐ Two sets of ten reps of close-hand push-ups

BICEPS CURL

- ☐ Four sets of twenty reps using a weight or resistance band that is comfortable. A good starting point here is one-seventh to one-eighth of your body weight.

SQUATS

Lower-Body Workout

☐ Three varieties, six sets as follows:
- First set: body weight only
  - Ten reps—standard squat
  - Ten reps—right lateral squat
  - Ten reps—left lateral squat
- Second set: add 15-pound (6.8-kilo) dumbbell or kettlebell (Goblet Squat)
  - Ten reps—standard squat
  - Ten reps—right lateral squat
  - Ten reps—left lateral squat
- Third set: use 20-pound (9-kilo) dumbbell
  - Ten reps—standard squat
  - Ten reps—right lateral squat
  - Ten reps—left lateral squat
- Fourth set: repeat first set using 20-pound (9-kilo) weight
- Fifth set: repeat second set using 15-pound (6.8-kilo) weight
- Sixth set: repeat third set using 10-pound (4.5-kilo) weight

LUNGES

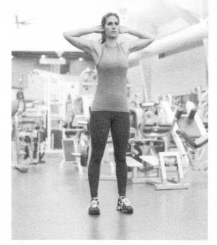
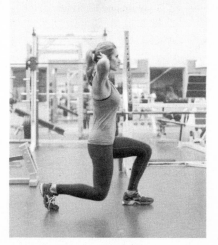

Figure 16

> □ Two types: hands behind the head or extended to the side at the shoulders for balance
> > • Forward—two sets of ten reps, one set landing on left foot, one set landing on right foot.
> > • Backward—two sets of ten reps, one set landing on left foot, one set landing on right foot.

The Martina Plan

Before I introduce you to the more intense Martina fitness plan, a word of warning: *Increasing the intensity of your workouts too drastically is a leading cause of injury.* Getting hurt typically sidelines you from exercise for weeks, even months—which will affect your weight, especially if you've been working out for some time.

So please, be very careful when increasing the intensity of your workouts. If 20 percent feels like too much of an increase, it probably is. Feel free to begin with a 10 percent increase in intensity, or even just 5 percent; both will increase how hard you're working your body and how many calories you burn without risking injury.

Remember this cardinal rule: If a workout feels too hard, it probably is. The most important part of any exercise plan is that the exercises are doable and safe, so you prevent damage and injury to your body.

MARTINA'S PHASE 1: WEEKS 1 AND 2

NO CHANGES TO YOUR ROUTINE

If you are already working out, keep doing whatever you're doing. If you've been taking it easy for the past few weeks, keep taking it easy. Keep your exercise routine exactly the way it has been for the past month. A change upward risks triggering adaptive thermogenesis, a stress reaction, and inflammation, all of which will sabotage your weight-loss efforts. A change downward alters your metabolism, and that's not good either. So, for Phase 1 of the Appetite Solution, *stay the course.*

MARTINA'S PHASE 2: WEEKS 3 AND 4

CARDIO: twice a week

Increase the volume of your cardiovascular workout (walking, running, elliptical, stairs, cycling) by 20 percent.

If you haven't been exercising for a while but would like to jump into the Martina Plan, shoot for thirty minutes of cardio at whatever speed works comfortably for you, leaving you energized rather than exhausted. Perhaps try walking at 4 miles (6.5 kilometres) per hour, or try running on the treadmill at 8 miles (13 kilometres) per hour.

RESISTANCE: three times a week

At this point, you can switch from your previous routine to the Appetite Solution fitness plan, focusing on shoulder stabilization:

- **Cable Internal Rotations:** Two sets of fifteen reps with very light weight (no more than 5 to 10 pounds/2.25 to 4.5 kilos).
- **Cable External Rotation:** Two sets of fifteen reps with very light weight (no more than 5 to 10 pounds/2.25 to 4.5 kilos).
- **Incline Bench Reverse Fly:** Two sets of twelve reps each; those new to this exercise should start with a weight as low as 5 pounds (2.25 kilos) and advance as tolerated; rest for twenty seconds between sets.
- **Upright Forward Shoulder Extension:** Using 10- to 15-pound (4.5- to 6.8-kilo) dumbbells in each hand, do two sets of fifteen reps, with twenty seconds of rest between sets.
- **Bench Press:** Three sets of eighteen to twenty reps with a weight one-third of your body weight or 30 percent less than you would usually use. Rest only twenty seconds between sets.
- **Goblet Squat:** Three sets of eighteen to twenty reps holding a weight that is one-quarter to one-fifth of your body weight. Rest only twenty seconds between sets.
- **Incline Bench Crunch:** Set the bench at a 45-degree incline and do four sets of eighteen to twenty reps each. Be sure to cross your right shoulder to your left knee and vice versa for the last six reps of each set.

- □ **Standing Biceps Curl:** Four sets of eighteen to twenty reps with a weight that is one-seventh to one-eighth of your body weight. Rest only twenty seconds between sets.

MARTINA'S PHASE 3: WEEKS 5 AND 6

CARDIO: twice a week

Turn up the intensity by another 20 percent over these two weeks. Don't be afraid to experiment with the preprogrammed workouts (interval training, incline variations, and pacing change-ups) on the machines at the gym to keep it interesting and to keep your body from getting used to any one particular motion. Or, if you're walking, running, or cycling outside, vary your route and pace.

RESISTANCE: Three times a week

Your goal is a total-body workout in thirty minutes, with no more than fifteen to twenty seconds of rest between sets.

Upper-Body Workout

SHOULDER STABILIZATION

- □ **Cable Internal Rotations:** Two sets of twelve reps with very light weight (no more than 5 to 10 pounds/2.25 to 4.5 kilos).
- □ **Cable External Rotation:** Two sets of twelve reps with very light weight (no more than 5 to 10 pounds/2.25 to 4.5 kilos).
- □ **Incline Bench Reverse Fly:** Two sets of ten reps each; start with 5-pound (2.25-kilo) weights and advance as comfortable, but never use more than 15 pounds (6.8 kilos); rest for twenty seconds between sets.
- □ **Upright Forward Shoulder Extension:** Using 10- to 15-pound (4.5- to 6.8-kilo) dumbbells in each hand, do two sets of ten reps, with twenty seconds of rest between sets.
- □ **Bench Press:** Three sets of fifteen to eighteen reps with a weight that is one-third of your body weight or 30 percent less than you would normally use. Rest only twenty seconds between sets.

☐ **Incline Bench Crunch:** Set the bench at a 45-degree incline and do four sets of eighteen to twenty reps each. Be sure to cross your right shoulder to your left knee and vice versa for the last ten reps of each set.

☐ **Standing Biceps Curl:** Three sets of fifteen to eighteen reps with a dumbbell equivalent to one-sixth your body weight or 30 percent less than you would usually use. Rest only twenty seconds between sets.

PUSH-UPS

☐ Two sets of ten reps of standard push-ups—hands at shoulder width

☐ One set of ten reps of wide-hand push-ups

☐ One set of ten reps of close-hand push-ups

Lower-Body Workout

SQUATS, SIX SETS

☐ First set: body weight only with hands clenched mid-chest
- Ten reps—standard squat
- Ten reps—right lateral squat
- Ten reps—left lateral squat

☐ Second set: Goblet Squat with 20-pound (9-kilo) dumbbell or kettlebell
- Ten reps—standard squat
- Ten reps—right lateral squat
- Ten reps—left lateral squat

☐ Third set: use 30-pound (13.6-kilo) dumbbell or kettlebell
- Ten reps—standard squat
- Ten reps—right lateral squat
- Ten reps—left lateral squat

☐ Fourth set: repeat first set using 20-pound (9-kilo) weight

☐ Fifth set: repeat second set using 15-pound (6.8-kilo) weight

☐ Sixth set: repeat third set using 10-pound (4.5-kilo) weight

LUNGES

☐ Two types: hands behind the head or extended to the side at the shoulders for balance (see figure 16)

- Forward—four sets of ten reps, broken down as two sets with each foot alternating as the landing foot
- Backward—four sets of ten reps, broken down as two sets with each foot alternating as the landing foot

MARTINA, BEYOND PHASE 3: LIFETIME

CARDIO: twice a week

Continue to increase your intensity during your thirty-minute workouts. When you feel you have reached your limit, switch to a different form of cardio. When you feel you have reached your limit again, switch again. Even if you simply alternate between two forms of cardio—say, running on a treadmill and riding a stationary bike—your muscles will benefit from the variation.

RESISTANCE: three times a week

Continue the workout from Phase 3, increasing the number of repetitions per set by two every two weeks. By Week 9, vary the order of your resistance exercise routine while still completing all of the exercises.

Varying Martina's Workout Plan: Avoiding Muscle Complacency

When you do the same workout over and over again, your results will stagnate. That's because both you and your body are bored! This phenomenon is called *muscle complacency*, and it's one of the most common and most unrecognized reasons why people burn out and give up on exercise. When our muscles adapt to the same workout routine, we get diminishing results in both strength and endurance.

You can avoid this problem by varying your cardio and resistance training workouts as much as possible. Change up the intensity, the order of the exercises, even the actual movement. For instance, once or twice a month, throw in a random yoga or pilates class that you don't typically take; that can be a great way to challenge your body.

Here are two examples of how to vary the old reliables, push-ups and squats, within a single workout.

Push-up Variations

Varying your hand position changes which muscles you use. First, try to do one set of ten push-ups with your hands located directly in line with your shoulders (figure 3). After a rest interval of about thirty seconds, move your hands to 6 inches (15 centimetres) outside of your shoulders (figure 6) and do another set of ten push-ups. Rest for another thirty seconds. Complete this new push-up unit by doing another ten to twelve reps with your hands almost touching each other directly under your chest (figure 7). This last position enhances the workload on another set of arm muscles, your triceps, as well as the big muscles of your chest and shoulders.

Squat Variations

Side squat: Begin at the same starting position as for the usual squat. Then, instead of squatting straight down, alternate squatting down to the right and to the left, each time returning to the starting position before the next repetition (see figure 2). Do one set of fifteen reps on each side. After a thirty-second rest, perform one set of fifteen traditional squats.

Lunge: From the starting position, step forward with your right foot and squat down so that your left knee nearly touches the floor (see figure 16). Do ten to twelve reps with each leg taking a turn moving forward. After resting for thirty seconds, perform the exercise in reverse, stepping backward with one foot and squatting so that the knee of that foot nearly touches the floor. Each foot should take a turn for a total of ten reps on each side. Feel free to hold on to a chair if you need to.

Part III

Hungry No More

Chapter 8

Solutions for Every Situation

Here's a scenario you might run in to: You've been following the Appetite Solution for a whole week, and it's going very well. You're pleased with how quickly your appetite subsided during your first few days on the program—it feels wonderful not being hungry anymore! You love how energized and calm you feel, clearheaded and full of optimism. You've even started getting a few compliments about your glowing skin and how terrific you look overall.

Then you join your work colleagues for your usual Friday-evening trip to the local pub—and your heart sinks. Mozzarella sticks, battered prawns, burgers on white buns with a side of chips, toasties grilled with tons of butter—what are you going to eat? And how will you feel, sitting there with a glass of soda water, while all your friends are tossing back beers and martinis and wondering why you're not joining in?

And another scenario: You're well into Phase 2 of the Appetite Solution, and you're so proud of your progress. You actually enjoy being hungry now, because your appetite shows up only occasionally—about half an hour before you're ready to have a meal or a snack—and it's a mild, pleasant hunger, not the overwhelming, ravenous sensation you used to feel. You're enjoying the exercise, too, which is making you feel even more energized and buoyant than you felt during Phase 1. To cap it all off, your clothes have started to fit differently, and you like the way you look in the mirror.

Then Christmas rolls around, and you begin to panic. The thought of sitting at the family table, looking at all sorts of foods that you can't have, with everyone pressuring you to eat, is horrible. Obviously, you don't want to miss a family Christmas. But you don't necessarily want to announce to everyone that you're trying to lose weight, and you definitely don't want to hurt anyone's feelings by refusing the traditional stuffing and your aunt's famous mince pies. How will you handle this?

And again: You're sailing along on Phase 3 of the Appetite Solution and feeling terrific about the three to five pounds (1.5 to 2 kilos) you are losing each week. With your new exercise plan, your muscles are feeling firmer, your whole body looks sleeker, and your clothes definitely fit a lot better—except for the ones that are now too big! You have more energy than you ever remember having, and you feel like there's nothing you can't do.

Then you have to leave home for a few days—a business trip, perhaps, or an urgent family visit, or a holiday. You know how to manage your eating and exercise plan at home, but traveling is a whole different matter. What will you find to eat? How will you manage on *three* restaurant meals a day, or when you feel like you have to eat *all* your food in somebody else's home? How can you continue your progress without being derailed?

Commitment, Flexibility, and Imagination

I'm always sympathetic when patients call me in a panic about a situation like the ones I just described. Whether it's restaurant dining, meals with the family, the holidays, or travel, these challenges can often feel overwhelming, especially when you are just beginning a new eating plan or even thinking about beginning one.

So let me put your mind at ease. In this chapter, I share with you workable solutions for every situation in which you might need a little extra support. I also give you some of my own favorite solutions for resisting temptation and sticking to the program while you transform your appetite.

I offer lots of specific suggestions, but basically, all my advice begins and ends with three words: *commitment, flexibility, imagination.*

☐ **Commitment.** Stay committed to the program. Or, as I often tell my patients, "Keep your eyes on the prize." Why are you doing this in the first place? You want to lose weight, right? You want to shed some of the extra fat that is slowing you down and affecting how you feel about yourself. Are you concerned about your health, trying to keep up with your kids, or focused on dropping a clothes size or two?

Whatever your motivation, keep it front and center in your thinking. Picture exactly how you will look and feel when you finally achieve the results you want. Imagine the obstacles that you will no longer have to face, and the triumph and good feelings that will be yours to enjoy. If health is your concern, imagine hearing the doctor giving you a great prognosis. If kids are your motivator, picture running across the playground with them or helping them fly a kite on a sunny day without getting winded. If clothes are where it's at, picture the new clothes you'll buy and how they will look on your body.

When your goals feel real to you, your commitment keeps you on course, because you can see for yourself that your long-term gain far outweighs any temporary satisfaction that you might get from having "just a few chips" or "only one drink."

☐ **Flexibility.** When the world doesn't make things easy for you, you can feel daunted and defeated—and I get it. But speaking as the guy who helps coach my sons' baseball teams, that's the point where I want to coach *you* to become more flexible as you search for another way.

Maybe your favorite pub doesn't have the perfect meal for your eating plan—but you can combine a couple of side dishes, or have a burger without the bun or a chicken breast grilled plain and served on top of a salad.

Sure, that holiday table looks like a minefield, with its white mashed potatoes, pies, and sauces—but consider having a protein shake just before you show up so that you don't feel hungry and you can focus less on food and more on family.

I know only too well how challenging it can be to travel, but maybe there's a small refrigerator in your hotel room (or you can ask for one) and you can bring some food items from home in a portable cloth cooler with a couple of cold packs.

When you have to make the Appetite Solution work in a new environment, things might not be the way you'd like them to be, but if you can be flexible, you can often mobilize a lot of help, support—and success.

☐ **Imagination.** Have you ever done word anagrams or jumbles where you have to take the letters that are forming one word and rearrange them so that they form a completely different word? The challenge is to prevent your brain from staying on the path that the first word lays out and instead setting it free so that it can rearrange the letters and think in new ways.

That "outside-the-box" imaginative thinking can be very helpful when you are taking the Appetite Solution out to dinner, to someone else's home, or on the road. Of course, every restaurant dessert is likely to be way too high in sugar, but maybe the menu includes a chocolate cake garnished with raspberries or pancakes topped with strawberries. In that case, you might be able to ask for a bowl of fresh berries for *your* dessert (my own personal favorite)—but you'll have to think outside the box to come up with such a request.

Sure, eating a family meal might seem challenging—until you imagine getting double helpings of the vegetables (*before* they are buttered—just ask!), bringing your own salad as a contribution, and scraping the sauce off the entrée. If you tell your host that you've got a medical condition that you'd rather not discuss, you can often blame everything on your doctor (go ahead, use me! I don't mind), rearranging a menu to fit your needs instead of feeling defeated.

That's the mind-set I'd encourage you to adopt—the mental and emotional can-do spirit and deep commitment that will help you make the Appetite Solution a roaring success. You can almost make a game of it:

"Now, how can I turn *this* situation into an Appetite Solution success?" Treating it as a contest or a game makes the whole experience a playful challenge, rather than a dreary duty—and you'll be surprised at how many people come forward to help you meet that challenge.

Now let's look at some specific solutions for restaurants, other people's homes, and traveling. Then I'll share with you some of my favorite weight-loss suggestions to give you even more support.

When You're in a Restaurant

These days, many restaurants have "light," "low-calorie," or "heart-healthy" choices that frequently contain fewer simple sugars and less fat. These choices, and sometimes even specialized menus, can indeed make it easier for you to follow the Appetite Solution while you are eating out—but beware. As we have seen, "low-calorie" and "low-fat" labels do not always mean "low in simple sugars." And the restaurant's idea of a healthy choice might not actually be so healthy.

However, many restaurants, even at the fast-food level, have options that might work for you or that you can make work with a little ingenuity. Here are some guidelines to make the process easier:

☐ **Be prepared to explain and to negotiate.** The nicer you are to the waiters, and the clearer you are about what you want, the better off you will be. Get the waiters on your side by acknowledging that you need their help and showing your appreciation: "I have a special medical protocol I need to follow for my health, and I'm hoping you can help me. It can get a bit complicated sometimes, so I really appreciate your helping me make it work."

☐ **Make your requests as simple as possible.** Giving the waiters an overview of what you're trying to accomplish can help them get on board: "I'm trying to avoid all dairy products, all white flour, and all added sugar or honey . . . and I'm trying to keep fat to a minimum. Here's what I'd planned to order—can you tell me if there is any milk, butter, flour, sugar, or honey anywhere in any of it?"

☐ **If the waiter doesn't know or isn't sure, encourage him or her to ask the chef.** There's no reason for the waiters to have the answers to a lot of your questions—but the chef will always know. If you thank the waiters for making an extra trip to the kitchen for you, they will appreciate *your* appreciation, and they might even start making suggestions or coming up with Appetite Solutions of their own.

☐ **Look carefully at the menu and be proactive.** Often, you won't find an existing dish that perfectly fits the guidelines of the Appetite Solution. So look at the food that's available and figure out how the restaurant could put it together for you. For example, check out the side dishes, and see what vegetables are available. Maybe there are some specials that come with vegetables, so even if you don't want to order the special itself, you can request some of the veggies. If chicken, fish, steak, or burgers are on the menu, you can always ask for a plainer preparation than the menu offers, and you can ask for low-fat cooking. For example, you might say, "I see you have salmon—can I get it plain grilled with no added oil? And instead of the white rice, can I get some of the asparagus that you're serving with this other dish?"

☐ **Be flexible (and I will be, too!).** If you're at a restaurant that serves breakfast all day, this is one of the few times it would be okay to have an Appetite Solution breakfast in place of lunch or dinner. Egg dishes with wholemeal toast, no potatoes, and some fresh fruit are often a terrific alternative, maybe even with a side dish or two of vegetables. If the restaurant has some peanut butter you can put on your toast, even better (but of course, measure it carefully!).

☐ **Make the word "grilled" your best friend.** Asking for your food to be grilled significantly minimizes your challenges. Grilling cuts down on the amount of fat that is used, and it also means that your food is unlikely to be breaded or fried (though you should specify this). If the restaurant offers grilled vegetables, you know they are likely to be fresher and tastier than steamed, and they are likely to have less fat than ones that are sautéed. Grilling meat, fish, or chicken means that the food will not be fried, and again, you can ask the restaurant to use as little oil as possible.

☐ **Ask for simple oil and vinegar for your salad instead of salad dressing.** Why get into a whole song and dance about whether there is honey in the citrus vinaigrette or sugar in the Asian sweet-and-sour dressing when you can just ask for the fixings and dress your own salad? That way you can also measure out the amounts and make sure you're not getting too much oil.

☐ **Focus on complex carbs if you get the chance.** You already know you're not eating white foods of any kind: no white rice, white potatoes, or white bread. Most restaurants will have whole-grain bread, some will have brown rice, and some will even have baked sweet potatoes and/or quinoa. (Avoid sweet potato chips, however, which are often breaded and in any case are too high in oil to be a good weight-loss food.) As always, be imaginative—look over the various dishes on the menu to see whether you can find any complex carbohydrates that might make it into your own dinner as you get the restaurant to mix and match. If you can't find any complex carbs to match what you'd be eating on the Appetite Solution that day, substitute another portion or two of vegetables. In a pinch, ask the restaurant for some sliced tomatoes. If the restaurant serves salads, you can often order a side of cucumbers and peppers so that you get some filling vegetables if it happens that whole grains or sweet potatoes aren't on the menu.

☐ **Maintain correct portion sizes.** No, I don't expect you to take your kitchen scales to the restaurant! But you can learn to recognize the correct amount of protein by sight. When you are following the Appetite Solution, you will typically be eating an amount of protein that is the size of your fist plus one half, or, alternately, the size of two decks of cards. Tell the waiter how many ounces you need (typically, 8 ounces/230 grams) and make sure that the protein you have ordered includes at least that amount; if not, ask for another portion and then take the extra home. You should be able to judge the amount of sweet potatoes, quinoa, or brown rice by sight. And you can't really overdo it with steamed, sautéed, or grilled veggies, so don't worry about them.

☐ **Take extra food home or send it away.** If you have been given a larger serving than the Appetite Solution calls for, portion out the right amount as soon as your food arrives. Then immediately ask the waiter to take away the extra, or you could ask for a doggie bag. It's very difficult not to overeat when extra food is right there in front of you, especially in a situation where you're more involved in the conversation than in your own bodily sensations of hunger or fullness. Make it easier on yourself by taking temptation out of your path.

☐ **Watch out for condiments!** As we have seen, condiments are sugar saboteurs. Please do take your measuring spoons to restaurants so that if you are having some allowed portions of ketchup, relish, or steak sauce, you can measure out exactly the right amounts. As you have seen, all that extra simple sugar can significantly disrupt your appetite, your metabolism, and your weight, undoing all your good work in a single meal. Why risk it? And to be on the safe side, do not order anything cooked in barbecue sauce. You are likely to blow out your day's sugar quota after just one or two bites.

☐ **Figure out your "go-to" substitute for alcohol.** You won't be drinking alcohol at all during your first six weeks of the Appetite Solution, and you won't be drinking it much after that. If you find yourself in a situation where everyone else is drinking, it can be awkward to focus attention on your abstention. Order a glass of soda water or your favorite diet fizzy drink with a slice of lemon or lime (just make sure to keep it to a single slice!), and probably no one will notice that you are going alcohol-free. This is one of those situations where others will follow your lead; if you don't make a big deal about passing on the alcohol, chances are that others won't either.

When You're a Guest

It can be tricky eating at someone else's house when you're trying to maintain an eating plan, but you really can do it. You just need a little creativity and tact.

You have a couple of choices for how to think about eating as a guest. You can ask your host to accommodate your diet by explaining that you're trying to eat very simply—no sauce, no frying, no white food, lots of protein and vegetables. If you're comfortable making these requests known ahead of time, that makes it easier for you, especially if you offer to bring a salad and/or some berries for all the guests to share.

Alternately, you can let your host know when you arrive that you're following a special medical protocol and that you're trying to eat very simply. At that point, you can ask for food without butter or sauce or simply scrape breading and sauces off fish and meats.

If you're unsure about what dinner will be, have a protein shake about half an hour before you start eating. Take it with you, if necessary, and have it just as you arrive. You'll be sure to get your required protein intake, and you'll be way less hungry during the meal, which gives you more leeway to pick and choose the food according to your plan.

Dessert can be a challenge. Unlike at a restaurant, where you can often order a dish of berries, the desserts offered to you in people's homes are unlikely to contain anything even remotely healthy, and they are virtually guaranteed to be loaded with sugar. You know all the sugar traps by now, including the seemingly healthy or "diet-friendly" choices like canned fruit, applesauce, frozen yogurt, and sorbet. Still, if the dessert really appeals to you, and you have to sit at the table while everyone else is eating it, that can feel like a cruel and unusual punishment.

The solution? Make sure you load up on protein at dinner, and bring another protein shake with you so that if necessary, you can have a second shake after dinner in place of dessert. If you like, mix this second shake ahead of time and throw in some sugar-free chocolate or strawberry syrup. If you load up with protein, you really won't have room to eat anything else, no matter how good it looks.

Many of my patients have told me about another common issue that perhaps you will face as well. They say that their families or other people in their lives are not always completely supportive of their efforts to diet, teasing them, dismissing their efforts, or questioning the rules of the Appetite Solution.

If you encounter a similar challenge, I encourage you to stick to your guns. If people are genuinely interested in what you're doing, go ahead and tell them about adaptive thermogenesis, blood sugar imbalances, and the way simple sugars lurk in the most unexpected places. Otherwise, keep it simple. Tell them you are following a medical protocol that you think will be important for your health and that you trust this approach. Then do what you can to change the subject.

People are often not sure how to handle it when a friend, family member, or loved one makes big changes in their lives. And some people actually feel threatened when a loved one makes a healthy change if they themselves are not yet ready to make that change. Let that be their problem, not yours. Be proud that you are taking such important steps to improve your life, keep unsupportive people at a polite distance, and welcome all the genuine support you can get.

When You Are Traveling

When you're traveling, you want to add a fourth term to "commitment, flexibility, and imagination": *planning*. Thinking ahead and looking out for the resources that will enable you to stay on your eating plan can help you make the Appetite Solution a success no matter where you are.

Here are some ideas that might help:

☐ **Take advantage of hotel refrigerators.** Even if a refrigerator doesn't come with the room, you can almost always ask for one— or ask to use one that they usually have available elsewhere. If you tell them that it's for medical reasons—which it is!—they will rarely charge you extra for it. When you make reservations, you will often see that a refrigerator is not "guaranteed," but you can almost always get one.

☐ **Invest in a portable cloth cooler and a couple of ice packs.** You can take with you some of the foods that will make it easier to maintain your eating plan: berries and/or apples; coconut milk or almond milk; perhaps some Greek yogurt, sliced turkey, or other portable protein sources. Individual servings of tuna, powdered protein shakes, and a plastic shake bottle can also be great travel resources. Look at the Appetite Solution menus in chapter 5 and take whatever foods are most portable and easiest to prepare.

☐ **Do some advance research.** Go online and find out which restaurants are near your hotel. You can usually check out their menus and know ahead of time what they offer that fits the Appetite Solution. If you'll be eating with clients and don't want to have the whole "What fits on my diet?" conversation in front of them, call the restaurant ahead of time and have that conversation over the phone. Then when you sit down, you can tell the waiter exactly what you want with the confidence that you'll be able to take care of that part of the meal quickly and easily and then move on to business.

My Favorite Tips for Losing Weight and Transforming Your Appetite

After more than a decade and thousands of patients, I've learned a lot about how to support your weight loss and appetite transformation. Here's your chance to benefit from all those years of experience:

☐ **Brush your teeth after every meal, especially after dinner.** The taste of toothpaste and/or mouthwash will dissuade you from snacking and make it more likely that you will avoid that trip to the pantry. Food just doesn't taste as good after a round of brushing and gargling.

☐ **Set a timer for fifteen minutes at the start of dinner, and when it goes off, leave the room for at least five minutes.** You will be struck by how much your appetite declines when you take a break like that. The food will seem substantially less inviting, and over time you will consume fewer calories.

☐ **Drink an 8-ounce (240-millilitre) glass of water fifteen minutes before each meal, especially before dinner.** You'll feel full sooner, and you'll also quench any thirst that might be masquerading as hunger. But as we've already seen, avoid squeezing lemons, limes, or oranges into your water, because you'll have the tendency to squeeze more and more juice into your drink, eventually igniting the sugar cycle at the worst time—before your big meal of the day.

☐ **Eat your protein first.** A good rule of thumb is to eat two bites of protein for each bite of vegetables, including salad. While you're on the three phases of the Appetite Solution, I've planned out your meals for you, but when you're creating your own meal plans, make sure to consume some protein at the very beginning of your meal. Don't begin breakfast by eating fruit, and don't start lunch or dinner by eating a plain green salad. Make sure that your meal begins with the protein that will jam your hunger signals and support your sense of fullness.

☐ **If you have any sense that your meals are too small—unlikely during the Appetite Solution, but just in case—consider using smaller plates.** Psychologically, seeing your food fill the plate will help you to feel fuller.

☐ **If possible, keep problem foods out of your house.** Ask the people you live with to support you in your weight-loss efforts and avoid having snack food, fast food, and junk food in your cupboards and fridge. Remember that sugary and starchy foods set up cravings, disrupt your appetite, and wreak havoc with your metabolism. As we have seen, your goal is to cut back on simple sugars, and that can be very hard to do if you are surrounded by temptation. The additional toxins in many foods—industrial chemicals, additives, pesticides, hormones, and the like—are all inflammatory chemicals that make it even harder to lose weight.

Don't Focus on the Problem—Focus on the Solution!

The longer I do this work, the more impressed I am with the commitment, flexibility, and imagination of my patients. When challenges arise, they often find such creative solutions that I am simply dazzled. As you move on through the three phases of the Appetite Solution and beyond, you'll be inspired to come up with your own responses. Keep in touch with me and the Colella community via my website (www.drjoecolella.com), and let us know how you're doing. I look forward to hearing *your* solutions to every situation.

Chapter 9

Appetite Pitfalls

Most of my stories are about my patients and their weight-loss challenges, but this time, I want to tell you a story about myself.

As so many of my patients have said to me, I was *sure* that I was sticking to my own eating plan, and I *knew* that I was sticking to my fitness plan; and yet, somehow, I had gained an extra five pounds (2.25 kilos). What in the world was going on? I was supposed to be a weight-loss expert, and yet here I was, gaining weight. It was upsetting, it was frustrating, but most of all, it was puzzling. I just couldn't figure out where the extra calories could be coming from.

Now, I often make dinner for myself and my two sons, and when I do, that dinner always includes a large, healthy green salad with my homemade vinaigrette. I use lots of oregano, some salt, a splash of vinegar, and a dash of olive oil—all healthy ingredients. I make a huge bowl, and we all share it. My two sons have that healthy teenage metabolism that we're all looking to achieve, so they usually bring a pretty large appetite to the table. And I started to notice something odd. Every time they asked for seconds of salad, I'd get upset.

Why? You would think that I'd welcome their eating such a healthy food, especially when it's usually so hard to get them to turn their attention away from the steak and sweet potatoes and focus on the vegetables. And yet, every time they'd ask for more salad, I'd find myself thinking, "I wish they wouldn't do that."

I finally figured it out: If they didn't eat all the salad, I could finish it all myself. And guess what was on that salad? You've probably already figured it out: extra olive oil. I had gotten so used to making the salad "by feel," I hadn't realized that my use of the healthy but high-calorie olive oil had gradually been creeping up, from 2 tablespoons to 3 to 5 to even 6. I was literally using three times as much olive oil as I needed to dress the salad—and that's where my extra five pounds (2.25 kilos) had come from. I started using a measuring spoon again, and within the week, my weight was back where it belonged.

I share this story with you for two reasons. One, even a weight-loss expert needs to use a measuring spoon! And two, even a weight-loss expert can find himself gaining weight if he's not aware of the many dietary pitfalls that lurk around every meal. All of us are only human—including me—and as we have seen, our human bodies crave calories in their drive toward weight gain. Your body thinks it's doing you a favor by trying to put on some extra weight, because for most of human history, it *would* be doing you a favor. Now, though, in our time of abundance, you can so easily find yourself slipping in some simple sugars or sneaking in some extra olive oil. And then *bam!* The weight you worked so hard to lose is right back on your hips, belly, and thighs; and you've been so careful in every way but one, you can't figure out how it got there.

In this chapter, I'm going to help you find those dietary leaks and plug them—every single one. Some of these apply to your six weeks of the Appetite Solution, and some will be important once you're creating your own meal plans later on, both before and after you've reached your healthy weight. I'm going to show you all the sneaky ways you can end up slipping more calories, fat, starch, and simple sugars into your daily intake—usually without even realizing it—so that you can avoid the pitfalls that my patients, and I too, fall into. I'll also show you the temptations that can sneak into your path—and some creative ways to sidestep them.

Pitfall Foods: Sweetened Almond Milk

As its health benefits have become known, almond milk has become far more common, and some restaurants and coffee bars offer it as an alternative to cow's milk. That's terrific—unless it's sweetened. If you order an almond milk latte, ask the barista or waiter to show you the box or at least ask them to double-check whether it has been sweetened. More than one of my patients has been fooled into drinking a latte loaded with way too many simple sugars.

Pitfall No. 1: Other People's Food

You've just finished preparing a perfect Phase 2 dinner: grilled tuna with some tangy lemon-dill sauce, asparagus spears glistening under a tablespoon of extra virgin olive oil, and a romaine lettuce salad with black olives and balsamic vinaigrette. You know that dessert is waiting—sliced strawberries topped with unsweetened Greek yogurt. As you sit down to eat, your mouth is watering.

And then you look across the table, and your flatmate has just set out a big bowl of macaroni and cheese—and suddenly, that's all you want to eat.

You're seeing that mac 'n' cheese at a vulnerable time. After all, you're right in the middle of a new eating plan and you're still in the process of reshaping and retraining your appetite. It's not that you're hungry—the Appetite Solution has taken care of your hunger by Day 4. It's that you're hungry *for macaroni and cheese.* You might never have thought of wanting that particular food, but now that you can see it, and smell it, and watch your flatmate enjoying it . . . well, now your own meal just looks second-best by comparison.

Believe me, I get it. And I also get how easy it is to take "just one bite" of that delicious dish across the table, and maybe "just one more bite" after that.

The problem is that even if you did just stop at two bites—and often, that's harder than not starting in the first place—those two high-sugar bites are enough to disrupt the metabolic transformation you are trying to achieve. As you'll see in chapter 11, you will eventually be able to indulge occasionally, and maybe even be able to have a whole serving of macaroni and cheese once every couple of weeks.

While you are still trying to lose weight, however, consuming that many grams of simple sugars and starches spins you right back into that old sugar cycle of cravings and blood sugar spikes and persistently high blood sugar levels, all of which trigger high insulin levels, which in turn cue your body for fat storage. Before you know it, your weight loss has stopped and your appetite is back to its old ravenous state.

Don't let one or two bites of a high-sugar food trigger a return to square one. Consider the following Appetite Solutions instead:

Appetite Problem: Facing Other People's Food

Appetite Solutions

- ☐ **Ask the other members of your household to join you on your eating plan.** That's the simplest solution—and it might be healthier for your housemates as well! If you can persuade your spouse, boyfriend or girlfriend, flatmate, kids, or others to eat healthy food for six weeks and to restrict their "treats" to times when you're not all eating together, you never have to see any food on your table that you can't eat, and you won't be tempted to take a bite.

- ☐ **Leave the table.** That mac 'n' cheese is at its most tempting when it's right out of the oven, bubbling and hot. In even five minutes, it won't look nearly as good. And walking away from it the first time you see it is going to make it way easier to resist the second time you see it. Excuse yourself, go to another room, drink a glass of water, and come back ready to stick to your plan.

- ☐ **Focus on your own food.** So often, we eat without really tasting our food, never really concentrating on its taste, texture, and scent. If another food on your table seems to beckon, direct all five of your senses to focus on your own meal. Put one bite of tuna and lemon-dill sauce into your mouth and really concentrate on the flavor. Feel how your mouth waters. Savor the lemony sharpness of the sauce and see whether you can detect the green flavor of dill. Chew your food slowly—see whether you can get up to twenty chews per bite—and really notice how deliciously it dissolves on your palate and satisfies your taste buds. Ideally, you will have a wonderful taste sensation; but even if you don't, your mind will be occupied with other thoughts than those related to mac 'n' cheese.

Pitfall Foods: Jam and "All-Natural" Fruit Spreads

These are all great examples of the kinds of foods that people think "don't count." You cut back on the butter and the peanut butter because they're high in fat, and you know you're allowed to eat fruit, so what could be bad about a little jam, especially if the label says "all-natural" or "no added sugar." As you learned in Part I, however, these foods are full of simple sugars. Avoid them at all costs. And while you're at it, avoid raisins and other dried fruits—and any food that is cooked with them. Check out page 73 to remind yourself of how much sugar they contain.

Pitfall No. 2: "It Doesn't Really Count"

Because you took "just one bite," that mac 'n' cheese you tasted the other day doesn't even register in your consciousness as part of what you ate that day. You told yourself that it "didn't really count," so you didn't count it.

Then, the next day, you're at a restaurant for brunch, and freshly squeezed orange juice comes with the meal. It looks so good when the waiter brings it, you don't have the heart to send it back. But it's "just this once," so you don't count the orange juice either.

The day after that, your friend is snacking on crisps, and you grab a handful—just one handful!—from the bowl. Your friend rarely eats crisps, so you're sure that you aren't ever going to do that again.

Can you see where this is going? By the end of the week, you've added several grams of simple sugar to your daily intake, you've provoked a number of blood sugar spikes that in turn generated insulin responses, and you're starting to have those old cravings that you had thought were gone for good. Because you told yourself that each of your little tastes "doesn't really count," you don't really count them—but each one has an effect, and cumulatively, they add up.

Appetite Problem: Indulging Without Planning,
Never Considering How It All Adds Up

Appetite Solutions

☐ **When you are trying to lose weight, stick to the plan 100 percent.** I suggested earlier that you think of the Appetite Solution as a medical protocol. That's no exaggeration: I have gone to great effort to ensure that each meal and each day during your six weeks on this plan have exactly the right balance of proteins, complex carbs, and healthy fats to transform your appetite and boost your metabolism; and I have also carefully calibrated exactly how many simple sugars you are consuming. A few bites here and a few bites there destroy the integrity of the plan and make you vulnerable to weight gain and inflated appetite once more. If a doctor told you not to eat even a single bite the night before an operation, would you think, "Oh, just a small bite doesn't hurt"? Never! If you can approach the Appetite Solution with the same life-or-death commitment, your results will be much better.

☐ **Once you have reached your healthy weight, plan your indulgences.** You have a couple of choices about how to do this. You might say, for example, "I get this many extra sugars each week," and then make sure you keep a count and that you "reset the clock" each Monday morning. It's easy to lose count, though, and to start eating your "future sugars" early ("I'll eat this now and then *no* sugar for two weeks!"), so I prefer a different way. Pick one day of the week on which you will indulge. It can be a fixed day—Saturdays, for example—or you can choose the day each Monday morning on the basis of what's going on that week (maybe your niece's birthday party is Wednesday evening and you want to enjoy some of the cake; maybe the big game is Sunday afternoon and you want to snack on chips with the gang). But pick your day ahead of time, and pick your treat ahead of time, too. That way, you know you've eaten it, you know it counts, and you know when it would be wise to go back to the straight and narrow. (In chapter 11, I'll give you a more specific Protein Protocol for indulging once you have reached your healthy weight.)

Please Don't Swap Foods!

Another common pitfall is "swapping sugars," that is, believing that you can substitute, say, a cookie or a few bites of cake for some brown rice on the basis of calories alone.

As we have seen, however, this type of swap will set you up for weight gain, metabolic failure, and an inflated appetite because calories aren't the issue—sugars are. Don't assume you can have "a few bites of something sweet" because "you have been good all day" if the sweet foods are high in sugars or starches. Chapter 11 offers a healthy way to indulge once you have lost all of your excess weight.

Pitfall No. 3: Mistaking the Portion Size

As you saw at the beginning of this chapter, even I fell into this particular pitfall, and I don't want you to come tumbling in after me. I can tell you one thing for sure: If you are gaining weight, or not losing weight, when you think you should be, chances are that you're eating 50 to 100 percent more calories than you think you are. To avoid packing in the calories and sugars, you really do have to measure your food, particularly the following items:

- ☐ **Condiments:** Condiments are very high in sugar! It's so easy to add just 1 extra tablespoon . . . and then another . . . and then another . . .
- ☐ **Peanut butter:** I'll admit, I get this one wrong myself. Use a tablespoon measure—don't trust your eye. Your sweet tooth can easily persuade your eye that you need *just a little more* . . .
- ☐ **Cheese:** People think cheese is a terrific protein-filled snack food, and it is—in moderation. If you don't measure your portion sizes, it's easy to overdo. Figure out what a 4-ounce (115-gram) serving is of whatever cheese you favor—low-fat is best, especially because it will contain fewer hormones and antibiotics than full-fat

cheese—and then stick to a single serving per day. If you'd like to split it into two 2-ounce (60-gram) servings, that's fine, too. I suggest premeasuring your cheese into individual servings and wrapping each one separately so that you don't have to get out the scale when you're hungry; you can just reach for the cheese.

☐ **Butter.** Butter adds up quickly because you eat it in such small amounts and the calories are so high. Many packets of butter come with a ruler on the wrapping so that you can measure exactly 1 tablespoon when that's what you need.

☐ **Coffee creamers, almond milk, coconut milk.** Don't just dump these into your coffee. Measure them—every single time.

☐ **Salad dressing.** You already know why you, and I, need to measure this one! Again, you need to do it *every single time*, or it's too easy for the amount to creep up . . . and up . . . and up . . .

Pitfall Foods: Soup

Guess which two foods are often used as the bases of soups? Milk and tomato juice. And guess which foods are high in simple sugars? Milk and tomato juice.

Soup has a third appetite pitfall when it is made with cream. Then it's lower in sugars but higher in calories—and, possibly, in the weight-promoting hormones and antibiotics that lurk in the fat of conventionally raised cows.

Because soup is liquid, it empties from your stomach more quickly than a solid, leaving you feeling less full than you otherwise would for the same number of calories consumed. And when soups include white noodles, white rice, or white potatoes, you're getting all of those sugars—and yes, they count, even in the soup.

Finally, vegetable soups are high in sugars, believe it or not, for the same reason that vegetable juice is high: the cooking process liberates those simple sugars from the formerly complex carbs, doing the work that your digestion is supposed to be doing and making those sugars way too easily available to your body. Basically, you'd do well to pass on the soup.

Pitfall No. 4: Drinking Your Calories

You already know to beware of fruit juices, vegetable juices, soup, and alcohol, but let me add one more caution to this list of drinks: protein shakes. This is the *one* type of calorie that you *can* drink—but be careful when mixing your own.

In my experience, people significantly underestimate the nonprotein calories present in homemade protein shakes. Of course, you now know how much sugar is in skimmed milk and blenderized fruit, but it's surprising how many people think it's okay to add those elements to a protein shake, as if somehow the protein shake would take the sugars away.

A better option, and the one I follow myself, is to buy a pre-made protein drink. They have the correct amount of protein, are low in carbohydrates, and contain a very reasonable percentage of fat. Just make sure that they contain less than 5 grams of sugar, and all is well.

Ideally, refrigerate them so that they taste better, but in a pinch, you can carry a couple with you unrefrigerated when you travel or don't have time to stop for a meal. If you really don't like the taste, try adding 1 or 2 teaspoons of *sugar-free* chocolate or strawberry syrup—not "lite" and not "low-sugar." You can also throw in some of your favorite artificial sweetener.

Pitfall No. 5: "Non-Food" Sugars

We tend not to think of cough drops or chewing gum as "food," and a single boiled sweet seems like "such a little thing." But all of these items are full of simple sugars, and the cough drops—which seem like medicine—can be especially sneaky. Avoid all of these unless they are the sugar-free variety.

Pitfall No. 6: Hunger After Meals or Before Bedtime

You aren't going to feel hungry at these times when you're following the six-week Appetite Solution, but it might occur after that, when you're putting together your own meal plans and still figuring out what works for you. Luckily, I have some fail-safe solutions!

Appetite Problem: Hunger at the Wrong Times

Appetite Solutions

☐ **Check your protein intake.** First, make sure you have consumed at least 8 ounces (230 grams) of protein at the meal. If you haven't, have a bit more. Open a can of tuna, make another protein shake, or nibble on some sliced turkey if no more of the main course is left. Protein should always be your first line of defense.

☐ **Eat fruit after meals.** If you've eaten your full complement of protein and you still want more food, wait ten minutes after your last bite, and then have either an apple or a bowl of berries. If you're still hungry ten minutes after finishing those, have another apple, some more berries, an orange, or some tomatoes. All of these foods will help you feel full without causing your blood sugar to spike, and you are loading up on antioxidants as well.

☐ **Have a peanut butter bedtime snack.** If you are hungry at bedtime, have one rice cracker with 2 tablespoons of peanut butter. You can substitute another type of nut butter—such as almond, cashew, or macadamia—if you prefer. This volume snack will make you feel full and satisfied almost immediately. Don't linger in the kitchen. Go to bed after you have this treat; it won't show up on the scale.

☐ **Check yourself.** If you feel hungry, ask yourself this question: Will a burger, a steak, a protein shake, or a piece of fruit satisfy my hunger? If the answer is yes, then go ahead and eat. If the answer is no, then you are not truly hungry and your brain and hormones are playing tricks on you. Drink a glass of water, and move on with your day.

Pitfall No. 7: Too Many Choices

This pitfall won't come up while you are following the six-week Appetite Solution eating plan, but you might feel a bit lost afterward. If so, and if you still want to lose weight, create a very simple go-to plan and stick to it.

Once you know you have a healthy eating plan, a little routine can make it easier for you to stay on track.

We are inundated with so much confusing dietary information about food, it can be hard to know how to choose—even for those of us who think about these issues for a living! So find a routine that works and stick with it, at least until you've reached your healthy weight. Doing so will substantially reduce the opportunity for mistakes at the refrigerator or pantry door.

Here's one final suggestion for avoiding dietary pitfalls: Focus on the Inflammation/Appetite Scale of Foods in chapter 2 (pages 51–53). That scale makes it super clear which foods will stimulate your appetite and create inflammation and which will keep you healthy, energized, and satisfied. When in doubt, let this scale be your guide.

From Pitfalls to Plateaus

Perhaps the biggest pitfall my patients encounter is the classic problem of the *plateau*—the point where you seem to stop losing weight even though you have more to lose. For solutions to *that* problem, let's move from appetite pitfalls to the plateau pitfall.

Chapter 10

Pushing Past Plateaus

Grace sailed through her six weeks of the Appetite Solution with flying colors. By the end of Week 6, she had lost fifteen pounds (6.8 kilos), putting her exactly halfway toward her goal, and she was looking forward to losing the same amount again in time for the summer. During Weeks 5 and 6, Grace had been losing about three pounds (1.4 kilos) per week, so she expected to reach her target weight within six more weeks at the most.

But a month later, Grace's weight loss had slowed to only two pounds (less than 1 kilo) per week. Then, the following week, it had stopped entirely. Panicked, she called me for an appointment, hoping I could decipher the problem.

"Let me ask you a couple of questions," I began when Grace was seated in my office. "Did you bring last month's grocery-store receipts like I asked you to?"

Puzzled, Grace nodded. "Okay," I said. "Then tell me, what item do you buy most often? What takes up the most space in your pantry? And when you think about the past couple of weeks and everything you've had to eat, which would you say are your favorite foods?"

Grace wasn't sure why I wanted to know these things. But after years of working with weight-loss patients and their plateaus, I knew the answers would tell me whether she had fallen into a common weight-loss pitfall—or had hit a true weight-loss plateau.

Yasmine had been very successful following the Appetite Solution. Like Grace, she had lost half of her excess weight—twenty pounds (9 kilos) out of a total of forty (18 kilos)—by the time the six weeks were over. She had continued to lose weight steadily, and she was thrilled at how energized, clear, and optimistic she felt.

Then Yasmine's company announced a new round of layoffs, and Yasmine learned that she was on the list of employees whose jobs would probably be cut. During the same week, her boyfriend told her that he had a new job offer in another city and that he viewed the opportunity as the chance to make a clean break with his old life, including Yasmine.

Between the stress of anticipating a layoff and the emotional challenges of losing an important relationship, Yasmine felt overwhelmed. At the same time, her weight loss stopped, and she even started to gain a little weight. On top of everything else that had been going on, the extra weight seemed like adding insult to injury. Distressed, Yasmine called me to see whether I could help.

When I heard Yasmine's story, I knew she had indeed hit a true weight-loss plateau. Fortunately, I also knew that I could offer her a solution.

Phoebe had been successful with the Appetite Solution, too. She had lost a bit more than half her excess weight during her first six weeks—about twenty pounds (9 kilos) out of a total of thirty (13.5 kilos). She expected to be all done with her weight loss in two weeks, but the week after she finished the Phase 3 meal plans, the scale seemed to freeze in place. The next week, she began to gain a little again, which provoked an immediate phone call to my office.

Phoebe hadn't fallen into any of the appetite pitfalls described in chapter 9, and all her grocery lists checked out. Unlike Yasmine, she hadn't been under any particular stress—in fact, other than the halt in her weight loss, things were going better than ever.

"My husband and I are planning a trip to Paris next month," she told me, "which is the most romantic thing I think I've ever done! In fact, I'm so excited, I haven't even had time to eat!"

"Wait a minute," I interrupted her. "Phoebe—have you been cutting calories?"

Phoebe looked puzzled. "Well, yes. I thought I could speed things up now that I'm so close to my goal."

I shook my head. "I'm sorry to tell you this," I said, "but I think instead of speeding things up, you accidentally slowed things down."

Diagnosing Plateaus

Just about everyone who has ever tried to lose more than a few pounds or kilos has encountered the dreaded weight-loss plateau. I define a plateau as a point in your weight-loss journey where you haven't yet lost all the weight that you intend to lose—but suddenly, for no apparent reason, you can't seem to lose any more. Even though you are continuing the same dietary and exercise habits that have been so successful up to that point, your weight seems to freeze in place, and in some cases, you might even start gaining weight back.

What's going on?

In some cases, the apparent plateau isn't really a plateau at all. Grace, for example, had fallen into some of the common appetite pitfalls that you learned about in chapter 9. For instance, she had been buying a Greek-style yogurt that was low-fat but not fat-free. She had also gotten very fond of getting almond milk lattes at a local coffee bar, not realizing that the almond milk was sweetened. A check of the box revealed that every latte had 5 grams of simple sugars, putting Grace's daily intake well over her 20-gram limit. Finally, she had been cooking quite a bit with tomato sauce, which, she admitted, she measured "by eye." When we looked at how much tomato sauce she had been buying, I knew that Grace was going well over the allotted portions for the Appetite Solution, and adding to her sugars there as well.

So Grace had not actually hit a weight-loss plateau. She had been falling into some pitfalls—which she immediately corrected, and to her relief, her weight loss picked up again immediately as well.

Likewise, Phoebe had not really hit a weight-loss plateau either. But cutting calories below the 2,000-calorie limit I suggest for Phase 3 and lifetime maintenance, she had provoked adaptive thermogenesis, which, as we have seen, is your number-one weight-loss nemesis, after simple sugars. Cutting those extra calories had "frightened" Phoebe's body into thinking that Phoebe was in danger of starvation, and so a whole host of chemical reactions combined to slow down her metabolism and halt the weight loss.

Phoebe had provoked adaptive thermogenesis even further by cutting many of her calories from her daily intake of protein. Instead of an 8-ounce (230-gram) steak for dinner, Phoebe would eat only 4 to 6 ounces (115 to 170 grams). Instead of two eggs for breakfast, she would have only one. Instead of eating protein-rich foods, such as a protein bar or a piece

True or False Plateau?

Sometimes you only *think* you've hit a weight-loss plateau, whereas a change in your dietary habits is the true reason you've stopped losing weight. If you think you might have hit a false plateau, try the following steps to diagnose *your* plateau:

- ☐ **Look again at chapter 9** to see whether you have fallen into any of the common appetite pitfalls described there.
- ☐ **Look at your grocery receipts** for the past few weeks. What items do you buy most often? What new items have you begun to buy?
- ☐ **Look in your pantry.** What do you have the most of? What new items do you see there?
- ☐ **Recall what you have eaten during the past two weeks.** Which favorite foods have you consumed? Have you eaten more of them than usual or added any new favorites to the list?
- ☐ **Look at your eating habits.** Have you been cutting calories, on purpose or accidentally? Have you been reducing your intake of protein?
- ☐ **Keep a food log** if you aren't sure about the answers to some of these questions. Write down everything you consume for the entire week, including such "extras" as condiments, coffee creamer, and that squeeze of lemon to flavor your fish. See whether any of the hidden sugar saboteurs from chapter 3 show up frequently in your log.

of chicken, Phoebe would sometimes substitute a piece of fruit. Cutting calories alone might have set off adaptive thermogenesis; cutting protein virtually guaranteed that it would happen.

Adaptive Thermogenesis Rears Its Ugly Head

Although Grace and Phoebe had accidentally caused their own weight regain by changing the way they ate, Yasmine had followed her weight-loss plan to the letter. Her plateau was a true plateau. Many of my other patients run into true plateaus as well. Perhaps this has also happened to dieters you know, or even to you.

So what's going on?

To understand what causes weight-loss plateaus, you have to recall the many facets of adaptive thermogenesis that we discussed in chapter 1. Adaptive thermogenesis is a very strong actor that is continually waiting in the wings, ready to run onto the stage of your weight-loss efforts and take over the microphone. Even when you take aggressive steps to circumvent adaptive thermogenesis, as we do with the Appetite Solution, it still sometimes succeeds in rushing on and taking over, pushing your body to hold on to weight or even to regain it.

Unfortunately, we don't yet have a diagnostic test to determine with medical certainty that adaptive thermogenesis is at play. What you can do for yourself, however, is what I do with my patients: Follow the suggestions in the box called "True or False Plateau?" on page 236 and try to detect any possible change in your eating habits. If you can't find one, then assume that adaptive thermogenesis is causing your plateau, and start taking steps to defeat it once again.

Push the Protein, Round 2

At this point you won't be at all surprised to learn that your chief weapon in the battle against adaptive thermogenesis is our old friend *protein*. You can get past your weight-loss plateau the same way you lost weight in the first place—by pushing the protein.

As we've just seen, there are two possibilities here. One is that, like

Phoebe, you've unknowingly slipped regarding your protein intake. In Phoebe's case it was because she was deliberately cutting calories in an effort to speed up her weight loss, but for many of my other patients, they simply forget to focus on their protein levels. If you have been eating *less* protein than is recommended for you during Phase 3, all you have to do is bring your protein intake back up to recommended levels, and your weight should start to come off.

The other possibility is that adaptive thermogenesis has caught up with you and is blocking your efforts despite seemingly adequate protein intake. In that case, you need to increase your protein intake still further to overcome your plateau. Your goal is to consume at least 1.5 grams of protein per pound (or about 3.3 grams per kilo) of body weight, using the ideal weight that you want to achieve.

So for example, if your ideal body weight is 120 pounds (54.4 kilos), you should be consuming at least 180 grams of protein each day:

$$120 \text{ (pounds)} \times 1.5 \text{ (grams)} = 180 \text{ (grams)}$$

Your first step, then, is to review your current daily protein intake. Are you consuming the right amount? Check out the table for some help in figuring that out.

Common Protein Sources: How Much Protein Do They Contain?	
Food	Protein (g)
8 oz. (230 g) steak	46
8 oz. (230 g) chicken	42.5
8 oz. (230 g) salmon	45
8 oz. (230 g) tuna	52
8 oz. (230 g) cod	35
8 oz. (230 g) low-fat (1%) cottage cheese	39
4 ounces (115 g) cheese	25
Two eggs	12

If your protein intake is falling short of the mark, you can use a protein supplement to make up the difference. Although you can find "protein shots"—highly concentrated liquids that are full of protein—I recommend protein shakes instead. Shakes include additional vitamins and minerals that boost their nutritional value, and they are often the best-tasting and the most convenient option available.

Is there an optimal way to time when to drink a protein shake? I've thought about this quite a bit and after careful consideration, I think it's really up to you. You know when you're most hungry and most in need of a pick-me-up. Go with your own instincts, trusting your body to help you find the right time.

How to Select a Protein Shake

- ☐ Make sure it has less than 5 grams of sugar.
- ☐ Make sure it has enough grams of protein to help you hit your mark.
- ☐ Try to get a shake with the most vitamins and nutrients added.
- ☐ After those three criteria have been met, go for taste and convenience.
- ☐ Feel free to add some artificial sweetener to your shake, or a couple teaspoons of sugar-free (not "lite" or "low-sugar") chocolate or strawberry syrup.

Protein Versus Plateau

The great news about the protein solution is how quickly it begins to work. Within a week of your protein push, you should see some movement in the scale, other than the normal fluctuations in water weight that inevitably happen over the course of every three or four days.

My advice is to weigh yourself once on the day you begin your protein push and then to stay away from the scale for the next seven days. You don't need to watch your weight fluctuate; you want to see forward movement, and you are most likely to see that after you've given your metabolism a chance to respond.

If you're comfortable maintaining this higher intake of protein, I recommend doing so until you've reached your target weight. That will give you the best shot of foiling adaptive thermogenesis a second time and sailing on to your ultimate weight-loss goal.

Set a Healthy Target

Another possible reason for apparently hitting a weight-loss plateau is that you have in fact lost a healthy amount of weight. In our celebrity culture, with its overvaluation of rail-thin models and surgically altered stars, it can be hard to develop realistic ideas about what your own body is supposed to look like when it's not airbrushed or tummy-tucked but just a real-life body.

My patient Chloe ran into this problem. At five feet six inches (1.68 metres) tall, she had her heart set on getting down to a goal weight of 105 pounds (47.5 kilos). When she stopped shedding fat at 115 pounds (52 kilos), she insisted that she had hit a plateau. I asked her where she had ever gotten the idea that 105 pounds (47.5 kilos) was the correct weight for her height, and she seemed surprised that I had even asked.

"Everybody knows that's the healthy weight," she kept insisting, and when I asked for more details, she reeled off a list of TV stars and models whose weights had been published in various celebrity magazines. With her big bones and athletic frame, Chloe was never going to reach 105 pounds (47.5 kilos) unless she starved herself to the point where her body was consuming its own muscle—and at that point, I told her, she would look nothing like the celebrities she envied.

Chloe eventually came to terms with her own particular size and shape and learned to enjoy how strong and powerful she felt when she worked out. She embraced her healthy target weight and let go of the unrealistic one. It can be hard to view your own body realistically in a media culture sustained by anorexic celebrities, plastic surgery, and chronically underweight film stars. The reward is well worth it, however, when you come to embrace your own healthy target weight—and then, through the Appetite Solution, achieve it.

Staying Safe and Healthy

If you increase your protein intake as I am suggesting, you should take two key steps to ensure your health and safety:

☐ Stay very well hydrated, making sure that you consume at least 68 fluid ounces (about 2 litres) of liquid each day.

☐ Confirm with your doctor that you don't have any form of kidney disease. If your kidneys are challenged, they're going to have a hard time handling all that protein, so make sure they are in good shape. You are especially at risk for kidney disease if you have longstanding hypertension (high blood pressure) and/or any form of diabetes.

Push the Push-ups

Along with or instead of upping your protein intake, you can also increase the intensity, frequency, or duration of your exercise. If you'd like to take that route, here's the formula I suggest:

☐ **Increase your cardio training by 20 percent**—which means going 20 percent farther if you walk, swim, or bike; moving for 20 percent longer in any form of cardio training; or, if you're using a gym machine, upping the intensity by 20 percent.

☐ **Increase your resistance training by 20 percent**—which means *only* increasing the number of your reps by that amount. DO NOT increase the amount of weight you use by *any* amount, which could put you at risk for strain or injury. That stressor could foil your weight-loss efforts both by inflaming your system and potentially by keeping you away from the gym. Research shows that you lose just as much weight and burn the same amount of calories by doing more reps, so stick to the safer path.

If you exercise five days a week, you should see results from your increased exercise within one week. If you exercise fewer days, say three, you'll probably need two weeks of increased exertion to see results.

Either way, as soon as the scale starts to move down again, drop back to your previous level of exercise. You don't want to accustom your body to a higher-than-usual level of exercise and make that your "new normal." Staying permanently at the higher level will only train your metabolism to expect that level of activity all the time. Then, if you run into adaptive thermogenesis again, you will have nowhere to go. And if you set your exercise floor too high, then any time you have to cut back—because of illness, injury, busyness, or advancing age—you risk gaining weight. Pick a level of exertion you can comfortably live with and increase it only temporarily, when your metabolism needs a bit of a boost.

Stress-Induced Plateaus

Sometimes a plateau is triggered by an increase in stress and/or inflammation. As we saw in chapter 1, stressors can be psychological, physical, or both, and inflammation can result from a variety of factors. Both stress and inflammation trigger your body to hold on to weight, to store fat, and to resist all attempts at boosting your metabolism.

Plateau Triggers: Stress and Inflammation

Psychological
- Romance/relationship challenges
- Trouble at work: deadlines; layoffs; difficult boss, co-workers, or employees
- Major life changes: a move, a breakup, living with someone new, expecting a baby
- A death or major illness of a loved one
- Troubles with one or more children
- A parent's illness or aging
- Financial worries

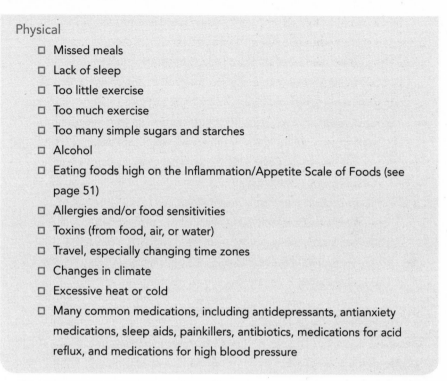

Physical

- ☐ Missed meals
- ☐ Lack of sleep
- ☐ Too little exercise
- ☐ Too much exercise
- ☐ Too many simple sugars and starches
- ☐ Alcohol
- ☐ Eating foods high on the Inflammation/Appetite Scale of Foods (see page 51)
- ☐ Allergies and/or food sensitivities
- ☐ Toxins (from food, air, or water)
- ☐ Travel, especially changing time zones
- ☐ Changes in climate
- ☐ Excessive heat or cold
- ☐ Many common medications, including antidepressants, antianxiety medications, sleep aids, painkillers, antibiotics, medications for acid reflux, and medications for high blood pressure

As we saw earlier, Yasmine had a stress-induced plateau. The double whammy of trouble at work and trouble at home combined to undermine her weight-loss efforts. I later discovered that Yasmine's doctor had prescribed an antidepressant and a sleep aid to help her through her difficult time. I believe these new medications also interfered with Yasmine's weight loss through subtly increasing her appetite.

If you think your plateau has been brought on by stress, or if you suspect it might be, take the following steps:

1. **Identify the source of your stress.** It sometimes can be challenging to figure out what has changed in your life—what new element, physical or psychological, is stressing your body. If you can identify your stressor, however, you can take steps to alleviate that stress, or at least to cope with it more effectively.

2. **Change whatever you can.** If your stress is caused by something you have control over—such as insufficient sleep, missed meals,

too much exercise, or too little exercise—then correcting the problem will likely make a significant difference. You can feel free to adopt the Protein Protocol that I suggest in chapter 11, but it will be far more effective if your stressor is not actively fighting to slow down your metabolism at the same time.

3. **Get support for coping with the things you cannot change.** If your stress is something you cannot control, as in Yasmine's case, you can work to change your own responses to the stress. Look for more emotional support, give yourself the downtime you need, or seek out other forms of stress relief: yoga, massage, acupuncture, time with loved ones, a brief trip out of town, or even the fifteen minutes of "me time" I suggest in chapter 4. If necessary, find a therapist, counselor, support group, or religious counselor to help you through a hard time.

If you are going through a stressful time, you can follow the Protein Protocol I suggest in chapter 11 at the same time, but be aware that it might not be effective until your stress is relieved, at least to some extent. Your body is powerful, and the stress response is one of its chief defenses. That is why working to ease your own response to circumstances you cannot change, or cannot change right away, is such an effective weight-loss tool. Even though Yasmine could not help being anxious about her job and sorry about her relationship ending, she could work to support her mind and body through those challenges—and that in turn could help her continue to lose weight.

The Medication Connection

What if your weight-loss plateau is the result of a new medication you have begun taking? This is a common trigger for plateaus, since so many common medications promote weight gain. Many medications also interact with one another, which can lead to even more problems for your metabolism.

If you suspect that a medication is at the root of your problem, discuss it with your doctor. *Do not, however, under any circumstances, discontinue a prescription medication without your doctor's supervision.* If you do, you could create serious medical problems for yourself—problems that would almost certainly sabotage your weight loss as well as potentially endanger your mental and physical health.

Again, the Protein Protocol I recommend in chapter 11, as well as increasing exercise, should work to combat any weight-loss plateaus that are the result of medication. You should also know that weight loss might alleviate some of the problems that produced the need for medication in the first place, especially if you are exercising regularly. Exercise can help combat depression, anxiety, sleep problems, and high blood pressure, and weight loss can help with all of these conditions as well as acid reflux. In some cases, losing as little as five or ten pounds (between 2 and 4.5 kilos) of excess weight can lead to clearing up gastroesophageal reflux disorder.

The Appetite Dynamic

Yasmine decided to find a counselor to help her cope with her stressful situation. Because her stressors were psychological, not physical, I thought some extra exercise might help to relieve her stress, too, so I encouraged her to boost her exercise for a couple of weeks. She also signed up for a package of five once-a-week massages, which she thought would help her through the worst of her bad times.

All of these factors together put Yasmine back on track to lose weight, and she achieved her target weight a few weeks later. She was surprised, though, that exercise had helped when at the beginning of the Appetite Solution, I had warned her away from starting a new eating plan and a fitness plan at the same time. Why hadn't this second increase in exercise triggered adaptive thermogenesis?

I explained that in most cases, it's calorie cutting, not exercise, that sets off adaptive thermogenesis. A new level of exertion makes the calorie cutting more problematic, but it's diet, not exercise, that is at the root of the problem. Now that Yasmine was eating a healthy, protein-rich diet, she could increase her exercise for a couple of weeks with no ill effects.

Yasmine was relieved to break through her weight-loss plateau and proud of all she had done to combat stress and improve her health at the same time. "Now I know that whenever I run into problems like this—either with my weight or with stress—I have the tools to solve them," she told me. "It's a good feeling."

Chapter 11

Enjoying the Metabolism of a Teenager

So now you've finally made it. You've been through the six weeks of the Appetite Solution and progressed halfway to your target weight. You've continued with Phase 3 for a few more weeks and reached your target weight. You've started the Appetite Solution fitness plan and progressed through the weeks to the point that you are exercising regularly, burning calories and building muscle. You can feel the difference in your body—the way you've become stronger, tighter, clearer, more energized. You have reached your ultimate goal: enjoying the metabolism of a teenager.

I promised that when you got to this point—when you had reached your target weight and sustained this new approach to eating and fitness—you would be able to indulge once in a while without gaining weight. And it's true—you can.

But there is one caveat: You cannot indulge mindlessly, without limits, because if you do, you'll lose all the benefits of your teenage metabolism. Consuming too many simple sugars too often will spin you right back into the sugar cycle again. You can consume *some* more simple sugars than you could while you were trying to lose weight, but not an unlimited amount.

In this chapter you'll learn exactly how far you can indulge and still enjoy your terrific metabolism, your pleasant appetite, and your healthy weight.

How You Got Here, and How You Can Stay

I admit, as much as I hate being the Grinch who denies you sugar, I also hate being the guy who tells you that it's okay to indulge.

Why do I say that? Because with too many of my patients, I have seen that when they view "indulgence" as their endpoint and their reward, they are tempted to let go of the Appetite Solution completely once they have achieved their target weight. Instead of viewing Phase 3 as a *lifetime* protocol and understanding the Appetite Solution as a *lifetime* solution, they act as though there are two different sets of dietary rules: one for losing weight, and another for keeping weight off. And the rules for keeping weight off seem to include going right back to the problematic behavior that caused them to gain weight in the first place.

A subset of this troubling attitude is the idea that you can fix at the gym the unintended mistakes you make with your fork—that you can eat a lot of simple sugars without consequences as long as you go to the gym afterward and work off the extra calories.

For good or ill, that's just not true. Eating huge amounts of simple sugars—going *significantly* past the Magic Rule of 5 and 20 (5 grams per meal or snack and 20 grams over the course of a day)—will sabotage all the good work you have done so far. Eating a high-sugar dessert—say, the equivalent of two bowls of ice cream—will overload your blood with glucose, provoke a flood of insulin, and set off a sugar cycle: a spike, a crash, and forty-eight hours of ravenous cravings for more sugar, which you will then have to use willpower to resist. The extra calories you take in far exceed what any realistic amount of exercise could burn off. And if you put in a massive extra burst of exercise, adaptive thermogenesis will cause your body to go into starvation mode, start storing fat, and ramp up the hunger.

That's what happens if you *overdo* the indulgence. But indulgence *is* possible, and here's how to do it right.

A Weekly Treat

Once you have achieved your healthy target weight, you can give yourself an indulgent treat once a week. If you are exercising regularly to get all the anti-inflammatory and blood sugar–stabilizing benefits that exercise can give you, you can splurge once a week on a food that contains up to 350 calories and 20 grams of sugar.

So feel free to enjoy one serving of ice cream, one piece of cake, or one slice of pie. Or perhaps you'd prefer some macaroni and cheese, a loaded baked potato, or an order of chili fries. One luscious treat—be my guest. And if you follow the Protein Protocol on page 251, you can enjoy your treat confident in the knowledge that it won't derail your appetite, your metabolism, or your weight.

Indulging During the Appetite Solution

- ☐ Once a week, you can enjoy a treat with up to 350 calories and up to 20 grams of simple sugars.
- ☐ Follow the Protein Protocol on page 251.
- ☐ Make sure you have achieved your target weight and are exercising regularly.
- ☐ Enjoy your treat all at the same meal, not spread out over a day.

One Big Treat, Not a Day of Little (or Not-So-Little) Ones

The first thing many of my patients do when I tell them about indulging during the Appetite Solution is to start bargaining. They want to know whether instead of one big treat of up to 350 calories and up to 20 grams of simple sugars, they can spread those calories and sugars over a single day, enjoying many little treats instead of one big one.

I wish I could say yes. But unfortunately, I have to be the Grinch again. Here's the problem: If over the course of a day you keep going over that 5-gram mark with your simple sugars, you're basically giving your body multiple insults that accumulate throughout the day. Instead of one blood sugar spike that comes and goes—and is modulated by the Protein Protocol on page 251—you get a lot of little blood sugar spikes. As a result, for that day, your blood sugar is persistently high, and in turn, your insulin levels for that day are high as well.

Those blood sugar spikes have the potential to trigger the sugar cycle in which you start craving simple sugars: a day's worth of insults probably opens the door to at least forty-eight hours of cravings. And if you give in to even one of those cravings, that elevates your blood sugar for at least another day, with another forty-eight hours of cravings. And so forth. Once you get on this ride, it's difficult to get off.

Meanwhile, with this "day of little treats," all that blood sugar is producing a steady elevation of your insulin levels, which, as you know, cue your body to store fat. You're basically reversing the fat-burning cycle you worked so hard to achieve. If you can tough it out through the forty-eight hours of cravings, you can get your insulin levels back down and, by the end of the week, reverse the damage. But if those cravings make it hard for you to resist more sugar, you're back on the path to weight gain, a sluggish metabolism, and an inflated appetite.

Basically, one day of exceeding your sugar quotas little by little is like a day at work when you are being constantly needled and nudged and given low-grade insults by a co-worker. By the end of the day, the cumulative power of all those tiny assaults leaves you feeling ready to explode.

Contrast that with that person coming up to you once at the end of the day and yelling at you for a few minutes. The louder, harsher encounter that comes out of nowhere and ends quickly is much easier to recover from than a day during which the little annoyances never let up. That day of insults takes on a momentum of its own that is far greater than the sum of all the individual incidents.

In the same way, subjecting your body to a lot of little sugar insults sets up a larger dynamic that is much harder to resist than the onetime response to one big treat. Once again, the problem isn't calories, it's simple sugars. And the issue isn't total number of either calories or sugars—it's the metabolic impact of whatever you consume. Because simple sugars trigger such a powerful insulin response, and because they have such an immediate effect on your appetite, their cumulative effect is greater than the sum of its parts.

Your Protein Protocol

So here is the Protein Protocol that allows you to indulge in your weekly treat without risking a return of the sugar cycle and its inflated appetite. Within two hours before indulging, consume 60 grams of protein, and within two hours after indulging, consume an additional 20 grams of protein.

That protein gives you a buffer that should cushion the effects of a 350-calorie, 20-grams-sugar treat. The easiest way to fulfill the protocol is to have a meal before your indulgence, and then a couple of hours later to have either a protein shake or another protein-focused meal. Obviously, you shouldn't eat a whole extra meal, so if you have your treat as dessert after dinner, then have a 20-gram protein shake before you go to bed.

The Protein Protocol

☐ Up to two hours before your treat, consume 60 grams of protein.
☐ Up to two hours after your treat, consume 20 grams of protein.

Enjoying Your Success

I want you to enjoy your new metabolism of a teenager and the weekly treat that it allows you. And I'm excited by the fact that every other hour of your week will be a lot more enjoyable now that you're at your healthy weight and receiving all the benefits of regular exercise.

At the beginning of this book, I told you that the Appetite Solution would bring you a whole host of benefits that you can enjoy every single day. Your skin will glow. Your hair will become thick and healthy. Your mood will lift. Your brain will clear. Your memory will improve. So will your sex life. If you have joint pain, you can expect it to decrease or to disappear altogether. If you suffer from symptoms such as headache or indigestion, they often clear up too. Many of my patients tell me they feel more confident. Most tell me they have become more optimistic.

Some of these responses, I know, are from the wonderful feeling of having pursued a goal and reached it, and some are from seeing clothes fit better and hearing compliments more often. But some are literally the result of good health—a way of eating and exercising that has reduced inflammation, rebalanced brain chemistry, stabilized hormones, and opened the floodgates to the body's natural sources of energy. When your inflammation levels are down and all your hormones are in proper balance, when your metabolism is humming and your energy is high, feeling terrific becomes your new normal, with all sorts of delicious side effects.

For Yasmine, whom we met in chapter 10, reaching her target weight also meant overcoming a lifelong struggle with moderate depression. By cutting out inflammatory foods—especially simple sugars—and reducing inflammation through exercise, diet, and the loss of inflammatory body fat, Yasmine made a significant difference in her sense of hope and well-being. The muscle-building protein she consumed was also helpful in providing the amino acids that our brains need to make *neurotransmitters*, the biochemicals used for both emotional and mental functioning. All in all, Yasmine's healthy new eating habits combined with her exercise plan made a world of difference to her.

Chelsea, whom we met in chapter 6, was the mother of two small and very active children. Thirty pounds (13.6 kilos) overweight and unused to exercise, Chelsea often felt as though she couldn't keep up. Once she was at her healthy weight and regularly working out, Chelsea had more than enough energy to play chasing games with her kids, take them to the zoo, and then enjoy a romantic evening with her husband at the end of the day. "I feel like I didn't just get a whole new body—I got a whole new life," she told me.

For Greg, whom we met in chapter 1, the prize was peace of mind and an extraordinary sense of satisfaction. "I felt like before, I lived life on a perpetual diet, always worrying about what I could and couldn't have, never understanding why I was so hungry, always feeling deprived," he said during his last visit with me. "Now, it's like I've been set free. I don't obsess about food—most of the time, I don't even think about it. I'm only hungry when it's time for dinner, my whole body can feel what's healthy for me and what I should avoid, and I don't ever feel like I'm depriving myself. I feel like I'm keeping myself full and satisfied, so I'm free to focus on other things."

One of my favorite patient success stories, though, is Maya's. Maya had always been shy and retiring, the kind of person who, as she put it, "hung back on the sidelines instead of taking center stage." Maya had a beautiful singing voice, though, and for years had taken lessons to develop it. The crowning achievement of her weight-loss journey was when she steeled herself to try out for the lead role in a community theater musical—and got it.

"I felt better about how I looked, and I guess I just had more confidence," Maya told me proudly. "But it wasn't more confidence just because of how I looked, exactly—it was more the whole combination of things: having more energy, feeling more positive generally, being proud of how much stronger I'd gotten and how much more weight I could lift . . . I just felt like I had decided to do something to make my life better, and I had kept my promise to myself and done it—I had succeeded. And once I had succeeded on the Appetite Solution, I felt like I could succeed at anything."

Maya's success and the successes of people like her are what keep me doing my job, and they are what has motivated me to write this book. I cheered for her success, and now I can cheer for yours. I know that your own version of success is close at hand, waiting to join you at every step of your weight-loss journey.

Recipes

This preparation can be used for any of the meat, fish, or chicken meals in each of the phases.

¼ cup (40 grams) diced cherry tomatoes
5 small black olives, diced
1 tablespoon extra virgin olive oil
2 x 6-ounce (170-gram) boneless, skinless chicken breasts
Salt, to taste
Pepper, to taste
Oregano, to taste
Pinch of garlic salt

In a small baking dish, mix the diced tomatoes and olives with ½ tablespoon of the olive oil, stir until evenly mixed, and set aside. Place the chicken in a separate baking dish and drizzle the other ½ tablespoon of olive oil over the chicken. Season the chicken with salt, pepper, oregano, and garlic salt, then bake for 20 minutes at 375°F (190°C/gas 5). Distribute the tomato and olive mixture on top of the chicken. Then bake for an additional 5 minutes at 350°F (180°C/gas 4).

TURKEY CHILI

This preparation can be used in any phase of the plan where chili is called for.

> 1 tablespoon rapeseed oil or extra-virgin olive oil
> 8 to 10 ounces (230 to 285 grams) lean minced turkey
> 8 ounces (230 grams) canned chopped tomatoes, undrained
> ¼ cup (40 grams) chopped red pepper
> ¼ cup (40 grams) chopped yellow pepper
> 4 ounces (115 grams) canned kidney beans
> ¼ tablespoon chili powder
> ¼ cup (30 grams) low-fat grated cheddar cheese

In a medium skillet or frying pan, heat the rapeseed or extra-virgin olive oil on high for 15 seconds. Add the turkey and brown the meat for 4 minutes. Mix in the chopped tomatoes, red and yellow peppers, and kidney beans. Add the chili powder, then simmer on medium heat for 18 to 20 minutes, stirring frequently. When the mixture is just about done cooking, sprinkle the cheddar cheese on top and simmer for 2 more minutes, until the cheese is melted.

SPINACH AND SALMON
Makes 1 serving

This preparation can be used in any phase of the plan.

    1½ tablespoons extra-virgin olive oil
    1 x 8-ounce (230-gram) salmon fillet, skin removed
    Salt, to taste
    Lemon pepper, to taste
    ½ cup (80 grams) spinach
    ½ medium tomato, diced
    1 cup (225 grams) broccoli

Coat a baking dish with ½ tablespoon oil. Place the salmon in the dish and season with salt and lemon pepper. Bake for 18 minutes at 350°F (180°C/ gas 4). Meanwhile, sauté the spinach, tomato, and broccoli in a skillet or frying pan with the remaining tablespoon of oil for 8 minutes on medium heat. Place the sautéed vegetables over the salmon and bake for another 2 minutes before serving.

JOE'S TGIO SAUCE

Makes 1 serving

This preparation can be used in any phase of the plan.

¼ chopped clove garlic
1 tablespoon extra-virgin olive oil
4 cherry tomatoes, finely diced
2 tablespoons low-sugar tomato paste
1 teaspoon lemon juice
Salt, to taste
Pepper, to taste

Thoroughly mix the garlic, oil, tomatoes, tomato paste, and lemon juice in a medium bowl. Place the mixture in a skillet or frying pan on low heat and cook, stirring with a spatula, for 3 to 5 minutes. Add salt and pepper to taste. Serve over any meat, fish, veal, or chicken.

TURKEY AND VEAL MEATBALLS   *Makes 4 servings of 2 meatballs*

This preparation can be used in any phase of the plan where meatballs are called for.

2 medium eggs
1 pound (450 grams) lean minced turkey
8 ounces (230 grams) lean minced veal
¼ cup (30 grams) garlic breadcrumbs
¼ cup (60 millilitres) low-fat chicken stock
4 cups (1 litre) Joe's Tgio Sauce (see recipe, page 258)

In a large mixing bowl, whisk the eggs. Add the turkey and veal, breadcrumbs, and chicken stock and mix thoroughly. Form the mixture into eight balls and place them on a baking sheet. Bake the meatballs for 25 minutes at 375°F (190°C/gas 5). Remove them from the oven and simmer in 4 cups of Joe's Tgio Sauce before serving.

MANGO SALSA

3 mangos, peeled and diced

1 red pepper, chopped or diced

½ clove garlic, chopped

1 tablespoon oregano

3 tablespoons chopped coriander

2 spring onions, chopped

2 tablespoons lime juice

1 tablespoon lemon juice

Stir the ingredients together in a medium bowl. Chill the mixture for at least 2 hours and then serve.

25-GRAM ISOPURE PROTEIN SHAKE

Makes 1 8-ounce (240-millilitre) serving

Use the scoop that comes with the protein powder to measure a 25-gram portion.

½ banana
½ cup (120 millilitres) skimmed milk
1 tablespoon natural peanut butter
½ cup (70 grams) ice cubes

Place all the ingredients in a blender and blend on high until thoroughly mixed. Serve immediately.

AVOCADO TUNA SALAD   *Makes 2 servings*

This preparation can be used in any phase of the plan.

- 1 avocado, lightly mashed
- 1 tablespoon low-fat mayonnaise
- 5 ounces (145 grams) canned tuna in water, drained and broken apart
- 3 tablespoons chopped celery
- 1 tablespoon chopped onion
- 1 spring onion, diced

Mix all ingredients together in a medium bowl. Chill for at least 30 minutes before serving.

SPINACH AND TOMATO OMELET

Makes 1 serving

3 medium eggs, whisked

¼ cup (40 grams) spinach

¼ cup (40 grams) diced tomato

1 tablespoon grated cheddar cheese

Salt, to taste

Pepper, to taste

Pour the whisked eggs into a medium skillet or frying pan. Once the eggs begin to solidify, place the spinach and tomato on one side of the eggs. Fold the eggs-only side over onto the spinach and tomato, and cook until done. Salt and pepper to taste.

BLUEBERRY WHOLE-GRAIN PANCAKES WITH OR WITHOUT EXTRA PROTEIN

Makes 1 serving

½ cup (75 grams) whole-grain pancake mix

½ cup (120 millilitres) water

20 grams IsoPure vanilla protein powder (optional)

½ cup (60 grams) blueberries (or any fresh berry)

4 tablespoons sugar-free maple syrup

In a medium bowl, whisk together the pancake mix, water, and protein powder, leaving the mixture slightly lumpy. Gently fold in the berries. Pour ¼ cup (60 millilitres) of mix per pancake into a medium skillet or frying pan. Cook at medium heat, flipping the pancakes when they start to bubble (about 1 minute per side). Serve with the maple syrup.

GRILLED OR BAKED LEMON PEPPER SNAPPER *Makes 1 serving*

1 x 8-ounce (230-gram) snapper fillet

1 teaspoon lemon juice

2 tablespoons extra-virgin olive oil

½ tablespoon lemon pepper

¼ teaspoon ground cinnamon

Place the snapper fillet in a medium baking dish or on aluminium foil. Season it with the lemon juice, olive oil, lemon pepper, and cinnamon. Bake the fillet at 375°F (190°C/gas 5) for 22 minutes, or grill it on medium-high heat until flaky.

SALMON SUSHI

6 ounces (170 grams) smoked salmon

1 tablespoon lemon juice

½ cup (65 grams) brown rice, cooked

1 tablespoon soy sauce

Cut the salmon into slices and pour the lemon juice on top. Then wrap the salmon around the brown rice as a roll. Serve with soy sauce for dipping.

HOMEMADE KETCHUP
Makes 1 to 2 servings

This preparation can be used in any phase of the plan, and it avoids high-fructose corn syrup.

4 cherry tomatoes, peeled
½ teaspoon red wine vinegar
½ tablespoon extra-virgin olive oil
Pinch of salt

Blend the ingredients into a paste-like consistency and use as needed.

BREAKFAST PITA

1 teaspoon butter

3 egg whites

1 tablespoon chopped green or red pepper

1 tablespoon grated low-fat cheddar or mozzarella cheese

Salt, to taste

Pepper, to taste

1 x 6-inch (15-centimetre) wholemeal pita pocket, toasted

Melt the butter in a medium skillet or frying pan on medium heat. Pour in the egg whites and cook for 2 minutes, stirring occasionally. Mix in the green or red peppers, cheese, salt, and pepper. Stuff the pita with the egg mixture and serve.

VEGGIE TORTILLA WRAP
Makes 1 serving

You can swap this recipe with any 400-calorie lunch in the plan.

¼ cup (65 grams) refried beans
¼ cup (30 grams) grated low-fat cheese
¾ cup (110 grams) chopped fresh veggies
1 x 10-inch (25-centimetre) wholemeal tortilla wrap
¼ cup (60 millilitres) mango salsa (see recipe, page 260)
1 tablespoon chopped jalapeño peppers

Spread the beans, cheese, and veggies on the tortilla, then add the salsa and the jalapeños. Roll the tortilla and serve.

Resources

Blenders and Blender Bottles

☐ The Magic Bullet Blender: www.buythebullet.com

This versatile and reliable multipurpose blender is great at home and on the go. Its functions include excellent blending for your protein shakes and making a perfect salsa. It also turns chicken into chicken salad in a jiffy.

☐ Blender Bottle, Inc.: www.blenderbottle.com

They make a terrific bottle that never leaks, as well as a tiny little bottle for making salad dressing on the go.

Kitchen Scales

☐ Salter Kitchen Scales: www.salterhousewares.com

They offer a variety of digital and mechanical kitchen scales.

Measuring Cups

☐ www.lakeland.co.uk

Lakeland offer a wide range of weights and measures.

Protein Bars

☐ Pure Protein Bars: www.pureprotein.com

They offer the perfect combination of protein and sugar (almost no sugar). The flavors are numerous and great tasting, and are everywhere in my house.

Protein Shakes

☐ Muscle Milk pre-made protein shakes: www.musclemilk.com

Great flavors with both a 40-gram pro series as well as a 25-gram option that are both gluten and lactose free.

☐ IsoPure Zero Carb protein powder: www.theisopurecompany.com

Get the 50 gram per scoop variety for the most versatility, and 0 grams of sugar.

☐ GNC AMP Extreme 60: www.gnc.com

It has only 2 grams of sugar per 60 grams of protein powder.

Sugar Free Items

☐ Hershey's sugar-free chocolate or strawberry syrup, available in specialist US food shops or from: www.thehersheycompany.com

☐ Frank's diabetic ice cream, available in most supermarkets

Supplements

☐ Vitamin D3

Take 1,000 IU per day.

☐ Vitamin B12 sublingual

Take under the tongue, 1,000 IU per day.

Vitamins and supplements can be found in most pharmacies and health retailers (www.boots.com or www.hollandandbarrett.com).

Measurements

medium apple = 5 to 6 ounces (145 to 170 grams) or 3-inch (8-centimetre) diameter

medium avocado = 2-inch (5-centimetre) diameter

medium peach = 5 to 6 ounces (145 to 170 grams) or 3-inch (8-centimetre) diameter

medium orange = 5 ounces (145 grams) or 2½-inch (6-centimetre) diameter

large orange = 6 to 7 ounces (170 to 200 grams) or 3½-inch (9-centimetre) diameter

medium banana = 7 inches (18 centimetres) long

medium tomato = 5 to 6 ounces (145 to 170 grams) or 2½-inch (6-centimetre) diameter

medium baked potato or sweet potato = 6 ounces (170 grams)

medium meatball = 2-inch (5-centimetre) diameter

small veal chop = 5 ounces (145 grams)

small scoop ice cream or gelato = 2 teaspoons

Acknowledgments

Extreme gratitude and love barely touch the surface of my feelings for my parents, Joe Sr. and Dolores. They gave me the foundation for the most wonderful life and no accomplishment of mine could have happened without their magic. Thank you to my brother, Dr. Mark Colella, whose expert vetting of my ideas and brilliant mind, not to mention his love and support, were essential throughout this project.

Thank you to my literary agent, Elizabeth Evans, who believed in me and this book from the very beginning and was a bright light even through the challenging times. To Gideon Weil and Nancy Hancock, the best editors an author could have, and to the fantastic team at HarperOne for all of your input and support. Thank you. To Dr. Donald Machen, a man whose brilliance is only outshined by his kindness, thank you for your inspiration and friendship. Dr. David Oliver-Smith and Dr. David Medich, my great friends, you have always had my back and have given me great counsel on things that matter, thank you. Dr. Elliot Smith, you are a phenomenal physician and a tremendous friend. Thank you for all of your care and kindness. To Dr. Daniel Benckart, you taught me how to be a surgeon and you have always been an inspiration. Thank you. Dr. Marshall Webster, you had faith in me and in this project since we met, and I will always be grateful. To Dr. Piero Giulianotti, a true pioneer in medicine and surgery whose landmark achievements in the field of robotic surgery have revolutionized the future of surgical care. Thank you. And thank you to Leigh Freno, whose technical skills and undying faith in this book truly helped to make this a reality. Thank you to Rachel Kranz, whose help with the manuscript was invaluable. And finally to my patients, who have given me the extreme honor to care for them and have provided me with an education that no curriculum could ever touch, you have my never ending appreciation.

Notes

1. Journel M, Chaumontet C, Darcel N, Fromentin G, Tome' D. "Brain responses to high protein diets," *Adv Nutr* May 2012; vol 3: 322–29, doi: 10.3945/an.112.002071.
2. Rosenbaum M, Hirsch J, Galagher DA. "Long-term persistence of adaptive thermogenesis in subjects who have maintained a reduced body weight," *Am J Clin Nutr* Oct 2008; (4): 906–12.
3. Mullur R, Liu YY, Brent GA. "Thyroid hormone regulation of metabolism," *Physiol Rev* Apr 2014; 94(2): 355–82.
4. Camps SG, Verhoef SP, Westerterp KR. "Weight loss, weight maintenance, and adaptive thermogenesis," *Am J Clin Nutr* May 2013; 97(5): 990–94.
5. Rosenbaum M, Leibel RL. "Adaptive thermogenesis in humans," *Int J. Obes (Lond)* Oct 2010; 34 Suppl 1: S47–55, doi: 10.1038/ijo.2010.184.
6. Rosenbaum M, Hirsch J, Galagher DA. "Long-term persistence of adaptive thermogenesis in subjects who have maintained a reduced body weight," *Am J Clin Nutr* Oct 2008; (4): 906–12.
7. Journel M, et al. "Brain responses to high protein diets"; Gosby AK, Conigrave AD, Raubenheimer D. "Protein leverage and energy intake," *Obes Rev* Mar 2014; 15(3): 183–91; Clifton PM, Bastiaans K, Keough JB. "High protein diets decrease total and abdominal fat and improve CVD risk profile in overweight and obese men and women with elevated triacylglycerol," *Nutr Metab Cardiovasc Dis* Oct 2009; 19(8): 548–54, doi: 10.1016/j.numecd.2008.10.006.
8. Symons TB, Sheffield-Moore M, Wolfe RR, Paddon-Jones D. "A moderate serving of high quality protein maximally stimulates skeletal muscle protein synthesis in young and elderly subjects," *J Am Diet Assoc* Sept 2009; 109(9): 1582–86, doi: 10.1016/j.jada.2009.06.3; Leidy HJ. "Increased dietary protein as a dietary strategy to prevent and/or treat obesity," *Missouri Medicine* Jan–Feb 2014; 111(1): 54–58.

9. Pennings B, Koopman R, Beelen M, Senden J, Saris W, van Loon L. "Exercising before protein intake allows for greater use of dietary protein-derived amino acids for de novo muscle protein synthesis in both young and elderly men," *Am J Clin Nutr* 2011; 93(2): 322–31, doi: 10.3945/ajcn.2010.29649.

10. Cooney GM, Dwan K, Greig CA, Lawlor DA, Rimer J, Waugh FR, McMurdo M, Mead GE. "Exercise for depression," *Cochrane Database Syst Rev.* 12 Sept 2013; 9: CD004366, doi: 10.1002/14564858.CD004366.pub 6.

11. Pennings B, et al. "Exercising before protein intake"; Markofski MM, Flynn MG, Carrillo AE, Armstrong CL, Campbell WW, Sedlock DA. "Resistance exercise training–induced decrease in circulating inflammatory CD14+CD16+monocyte percentage without weight loss in older adults," *Eur J Appl Physiol.* Aug 2014; 114(8): 1737–48, doi: 10.1007/s00421-014-2902-1.

12. Brenmoehl J, Albrecht E, Komolka K, Schering L, Langhammer M, Hoeflich A, Maak S. "Irisin is elevated in skeletal muscle and serum of mice immediately after acute exercise," *Int J Biol Sci* 11 Mar 2014; 10(3): 338–49, doi: 10.7150/ijbs.7972.

13. Saito M. "Brown adipose tissue as a therapeutic target for human obesity," *Obes Res Clin Pract* Dec 2013; 7(6): e432–38.

14. Weigle D, Breen P, Matthys C, Callahan H, Meeuwsk K, Burden V, Purnell J. "A high-protein diet induces sustained reductions in appetite, ad libitum calorie intake, and body weight despite compensatory changes in diurnal plasma leptin and ghrelin concentrations," *Am J Clin Nutr* July 2005; 82: 141–48.

15. Kellet GL, Brot-Laroche E, Mace OJ, Leturque A. "Sugar absorption in the intestine: the role of GLU2," *Ann Rev Nutr* 2008; 28: 35–54, doi: 10.1146/annurev.nutr.28.061807.155518.

16. Zhang G, Hamaker BR. "Slowly digestible starch: concept, mechanism, and proposed extended glycemic index," *Crit Rev Food Sci Nutrition* Nov 2009; 49(10): 852–67, doi: 10.1080/10408390903372466.

17. George TW, Niwat C, Waroonphan S, Gordon MH, Lovegrove JA. "Effects of chronic and acute consumption of fruit-and-vegetable-puree-based drinks on vasodilation, risk factors for CVD and the response as a result of the eNOS G298T polymorphism," *Proc Nutr Soc* May 2009; 68(2): 148–61.

18. Whigham LD, Valentine AR, Johnson LK, Zhang Z, Atkinson RL, Tanumihardjo SA. "Increased vegetable and fruit consumption during weight loss effort correlates with increased weight and fat loss," *Nutr Diabetes.* 1 Oct 2012; 2: e48, doi: 10.1038/nutd.2012.22.

19. Blom WA, Stafleu A, de Graaf C, Kok FJ, Schaafsma G, Hendriks HF. "Ghrelin response to carbohydrate enriched breakfast is related to insulin," *Am J Clin Nutr* Feb 2005; 81(2): 367–75.

20. Benetti E, Mastrocola R, Rogazzo M, Chiazza F, Aragno M, Fantozzi R, Collino M, Minetto MA. "High sugar intake and development of skeletal muscle insulin resistance and inflammation in mice: a protective role for PPAR-δ agonism," *Mediators Inflamm.* 2013; 2013: 509502, doi: 10.1155/2013/509502.

21. Blüher M. "Adipose tissue—an endocrine organ" [in German], *Internist (Berl)* Jun 2014; 55(6): 687–97, doi: 10.1007/s00108-014-3456-3.

22. Van Cauter E, Spiegel K, Tasali E, Leproult R. "Metabolic consequences of sleep and sleep loss," *Appetite* May 2014; 76: 60–65, doi: 10.1016/j.appet.2014.01.003; Guyon A, Balbo M, Morselli LL, Tasali E, Leproult R, L'Hermite-Balériaux M, Van Cauter E, Spiegel K. "Adverse effects of two nights of sleep restriction on the hypothalamic-pituitary-adrenal axis in healthy men," *J Clin Endocrinol Metab* Aug 2014; 99(8): 2861–68, doi: 10.1210/jc.2013-4254.

23. Page KA, Chan O, Arora J, Belfort-Deaguiar R, Dzuira J, Roehmholdt B, Cline GW, Naik S, Sinha R, Constable RT, Sherwin RS. "Effects of fructose vs glucose on regional cerebral blood flow in the brain regions involved with appetite and reward pathways," *JAMA* 2 Jan 2013; 309(1): 63–70, doi: 10.1001/jama.2012.116975.

24. Soenen S, Westerterp-Plantenga MS. "Proteins and satiety: implications for weight management," *Curr Opin Clin Nutr Metab Care.* Nov 2008; 11(6): 747–51, doi: 10.1097/MCO.0b013e328311a8c4.

25. Sobrino Crespo C, Perianes Cachero A, Puebla Jimenez L, Barrios V, Arilla Ferreiro E. "Peptides and food intake," *Front Endocrinol (Lausanne)* 24 Apr 2014; 5: 58, doi: 10.3389/fendo.2014.00058.

26. Gosby AK, Conigrave AD, Raubenheimer D. "Protein leverage and energy intake," *Obes Rev* Mar 2014; 15(3): 183–91.

27. Leidy HJ. "Increased dietary protein as a dietary strategy to prevent and/or treat obesity," *Missouri Medicine* Jan–Feb 2014; 111(1): 54–58.

28. Cordoso Fernandes Toffolo M, Silva de Aguiar-Nemer A, Aparecida de Silva-Fonseca V. "Alcohol: effects on nutritional status, lipid profile, and blood pressure," *J Endocrinol Metab* Dec 2012; 2(6): 205–11.

29. Nelson DE, Jarman DW, Rehm J, Greenfield TK, Rey G, Kerr WC, Miller P, Shield KD, Ye Y, Naimi TS. "Alcohol-attributable cancer deaths and years of potential life lost in the United States," *Am J Public Health* Apr 2013; 103(4): 641–48.

30. Sayon-Orea C, Martinez-Gonzalez MA, and Bes-Rastrollo M. "Alcohol consumption and body weight: a systematic review," *Nutr Rev* Aug 2011; 69(8): 419–31, doi: 10.1111/j.1753–4887.2011.00403.x.

31. Colton HR, Altevogt BM, Institute of Medicine Committee on Sleep Medicine and Research. *Sleep Disorders and Sleep Deprivation: An Unmet Public Health Problem* (Washington, DC: National Academies Press, 2006).

32. Brenmoehl J, Albrecht E, Komolka K, Schering L, Langhammer M, Hoeflich A, Maak S. "Irisin is elevated in skeletal muscle and serum of mice immediately after acute exercise," *Int J Biol Sci* 11 Mar 2014; 10(3): 338–49, doi: 10.7150/ijbs.7972.

33. Craft LL, Perna FM. "The benefits of exercise for the clinically depressed," *Prim Care Companion J Clin Psychiatry* 2004; 6(3): 104–11.

34. Deardorff J. "The afterburners: is post workout calorie burn real?," *Chicago Tribune*, 1 Feb 2012.

Index

About the Author

Joseph J. Colella, M.D., F.A.C.S., is an internationally recognized weight-loss expert, and robotic/bariatric surgeon. He has served as an Assistant Professor of Surgery at the University of Pittsburgh Medical School, Hahnemann Medical School, The Medical College of Pennsylvania, and The Drexel University College of Medicine. He is a founding member of and is currently on the executive Board of the Clinical Robotic Surgery Association, an international association of the world's premier robotic surgeons. Dr. Colella is one of the few weight-loss experts in the world with his level of surgical training and experience, which allows for a singular perspective on human anatomy, physiology and disease processes.